MDSAP

A Complete Guide

For All

Medical Industries

Second Edition

Online Certification
www.iscasc.com

ISC International
Vancouver, BC CANADA

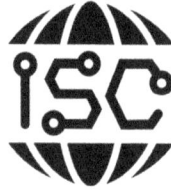

WWW.ISCASC.COM

ISC is one of the first certification
bodies to provide machine learning and developing and
applying **Artificial Intelligence** Technology in all
aspects of management system standards and certification
services globally.

Published by: ISC **International Standard Certification**
Vancouver, BC **CANADA**
Email: Info@ISCASC.COM

Ordering Information:
Quantity sales. Special discounts are available on quantity purchases by universities, schools, corporations, associations, and others. For details, contact the "Sales Department" at the above mentioned email address.

MDSAP a Complete Guide/ISC International — 2nd ed.
ISBN: 978-1-77899-004-5   Paperback
ISBN: 978-1-77899-005-2   Hardcover

Contents

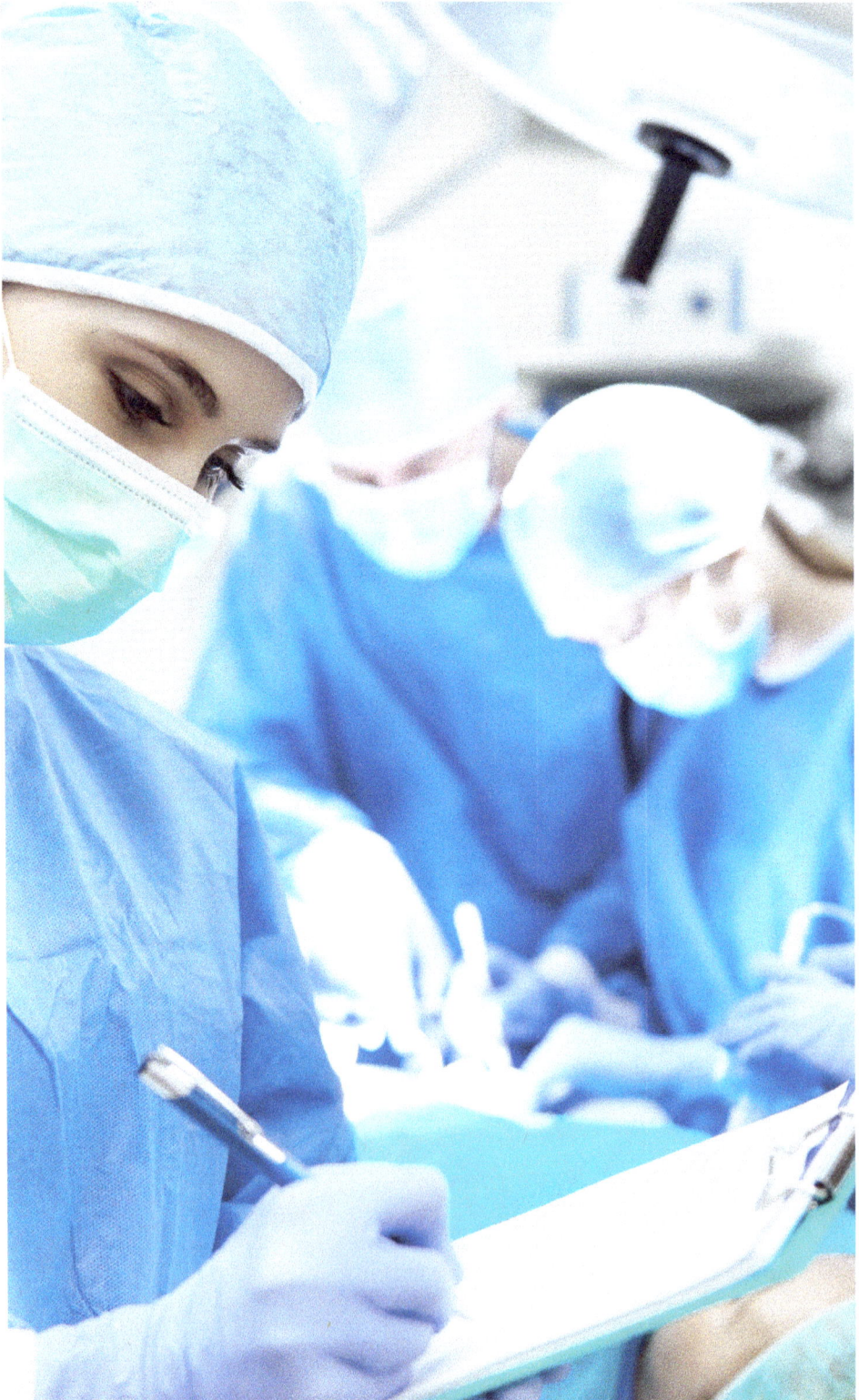

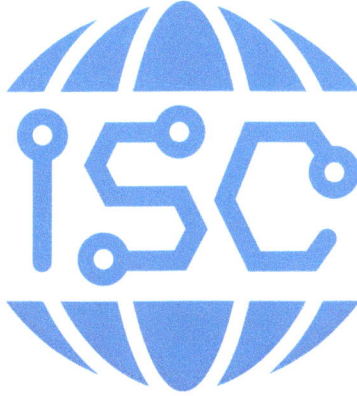

Every possible effort has been made to ensure that the information contained in this book is accurate at the time of going to press, and the publishers and the author cannot accept responsibility for any errors or omissions, however caused. No responsibility for loss or damage occasioned to any person acting, or refraining from action, as a result of the material in this publication can be accepted by the publisher and/or the author.

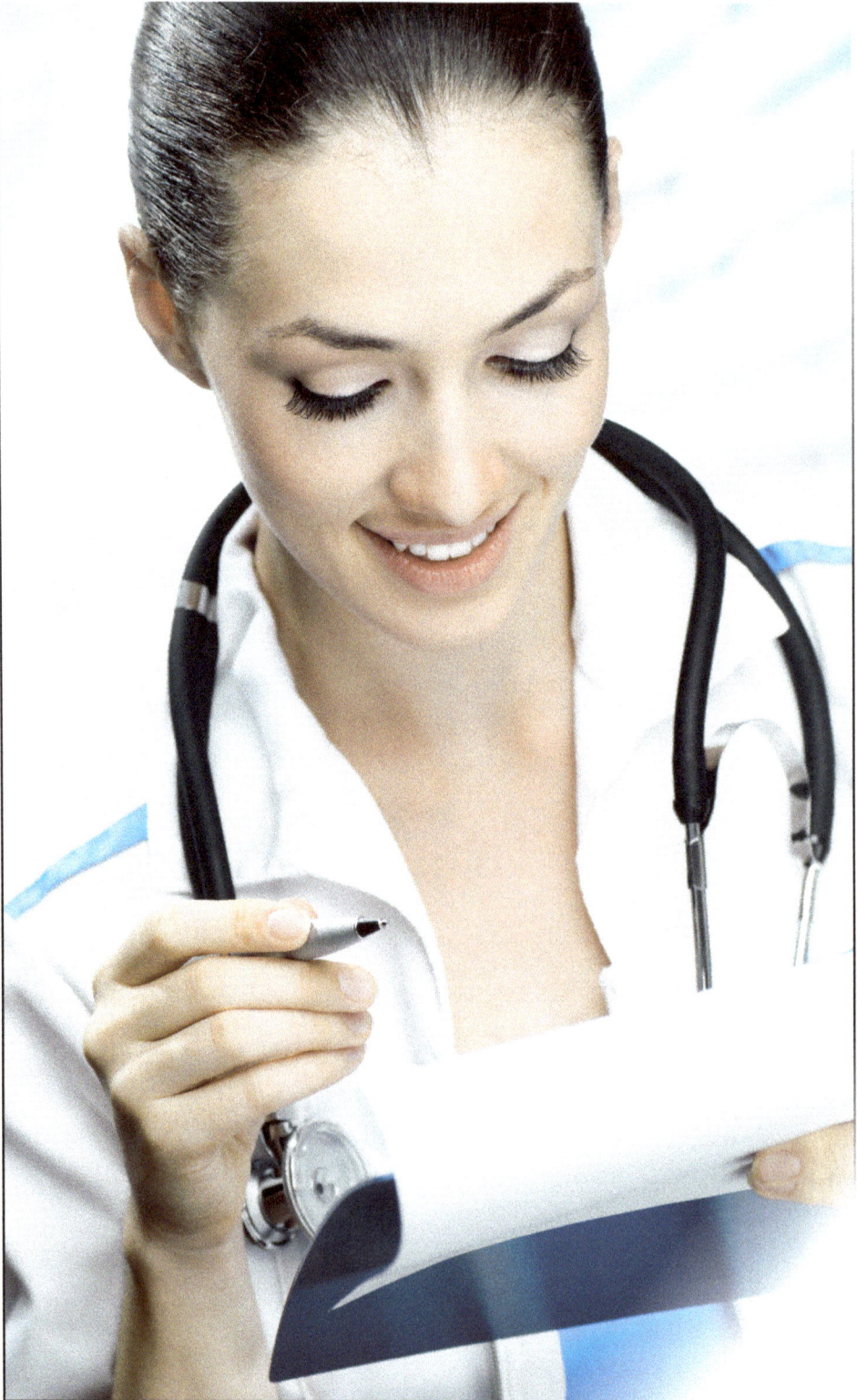

International Standard Certification

ISC is a certification body that Provides certification services. ISC Publishes different educational books and provides educational courses and certification services. ISC operates under industry-approved international standards and requirements and maintains integrity and impartiality while taking into account professional and public interests. International Standard Certification (ISC) provides objective evidence that a person or an organization operates at the highest level of ethical, legal, professional, and technical standards.

ISC certifies a wide range of professionals and organizations, including governmental entities, commercial businesses, and professional associations. International Standard Certification (ISC) certification programs are based on recognized national and international compliance standards that ensure domestic and global acceptance.

International Standard Certification (ISC) is the leading skill development and certification body for professionals and organizations compliant with the ISO/IEC international standards that form a unified system for evaluating and recognizing competent certification bodies worldwide. As a global skill development and certification body, International Standard Certification (ISC) is committed to ensuring excellent service standards delivered by those we comply.

ISO/IEC is renowned for its rigorous compliance standards – influencing our approach to certify professionals and organizations, so we can serve you and your organization at the highest levels possible and positively influence your business results that would not happen otherwise.

International Standard Certification (ISC) Certified Professional Certification programs' chief goal is to be market-relevant, consensus-based, support innovation, and provide solutions to global challenges. That means thriving career chances for professionals, and meeting and exceeding demands from businesses and their valuable clients.

What Made Us Decide To Help Professionals?
Let us tell you this. The shock of getting fired helped us admit three very important things that we haven't been entirely honest ourselves before: Large companies move slowly. Good ideas often died on the vine simply because they had to be approved by too many people. Climbing the corporate ladder is an obstacle to doing great work. We wanted to focus on getting things done and making things better, not constantly positioning ourselves for promotion. Politics and turf wars are an inescapable part of the daily experience of working for a large company. Frustration leads to burnout. We wanted to enjoy our daily work experience, but instead, We felt like We were running a gauntlet each day. It began to affect our health during working in happiness for all employees, friends, and family.

Why Did We Build The ISC?
We started the idea of ISC in 2009 with great knowledge of marketing, sales, persuasion, closing, e-commerce, and/or automated digital marketing systems. The more We learned, the more helpless We felt. For every great resource We found, I had to process ten other resources to figure out how to apply that resource in practice to excel on our own professional journey. We started to wonder: how much of what's out there —and there is a lot out there— We really needed to know. How could I separate practical business and professional skills from the dry theory and technobabble? We only had so much time and energy, so We started searching for a filter: something that would direct us to use skills and keep us away from the chaff. The more we searched, the more we realized it didn't exist — so we decided to create the International Standard Certification (ISC).

As of this moment, more than 5700 ISC Professionals, employees, employers, teachers, and schools, ... are actively using International Standard Certification (ISC) Services, publications, educational books, certifications, and Training to quickly get their ideas, products, and services out to the world!

So take a deep breath. It's time for you to unlock the blueprint of success as a professional and get to work.

Welcome to the International Standard Certification (ISC)

info@iscasc.com

Our Signature for your Success

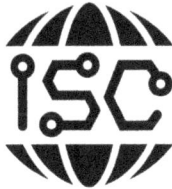

WWW.ISCASC.COM

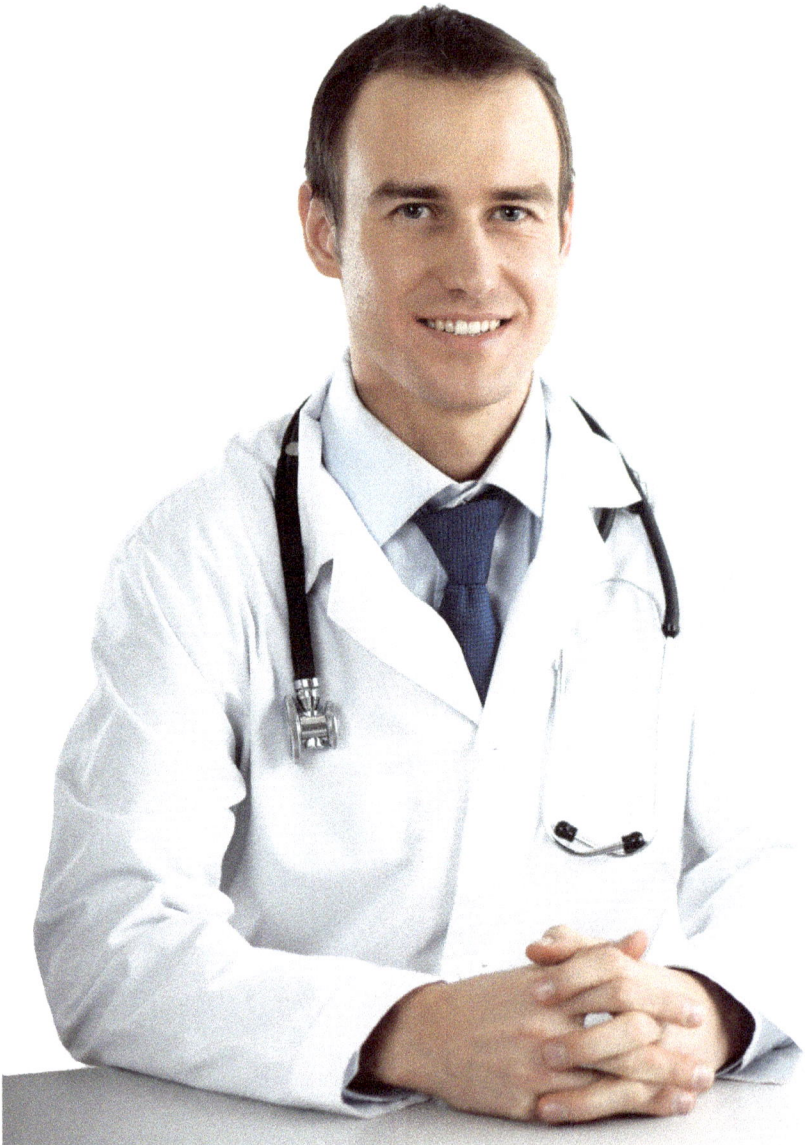

CHAPTER 2

MDSAP

MDSAP The Medical Device Single Audit Program is the single audit program that covers the regulations of Australia, Brazil, Canada, Japan and USA. These regulations use the MDSAP to verify compliance to the quality systems of their national regulations and ISO 13485. The intention of the Medical Device Single Audit Program (MDSAP) is to allow competent auditors from MDSAP recognized Auditing Organizations (AOs) to conduct a single audit of a medical device organization's quality management system that will satisfy the requirements of the medical device regulatory authorities participating in the MDSAP program.

Audits performed under the MDSAP program will be process based, focusing on several defined processes, a defined method for linking those processes, and built on a foundation of requirements for risk management.

ISO 13485 MDSAP are two different programs with similar requirements but they do not duplicate each other.

MDSAP has the more stringent requirements of the two and companies that are already certified to ISO 13485 will see an increase in the number of audit days once they seek certification to MDSAP. The design of the Medical Device Single Audit Program (MDSAP) audit process is to ensure a single audit will provide efficient yet thorough coverage of regulatory requirements.

These requirements include; Medical devices – Quality management systems – Requirements for regulatory purposes (ISO 13485:2016), the Quality Management System requirements of the Conformity Assessment Procedures of the Australian Therapeutic

11

Goods (Medical Devices) Regulations (TG(MD)R Sch3), the Brazilian Good Manufacturing Practices (RDC ANVISA 16/2013), the Japanese Ordinance on Standards for Manufacturing Control and Quality Control of Medical Devices and In Vitro Diagnostic Reagents (MHLW Ministerial Ordinance No. 169), the Quality System Regulation (21 CFR Part 820), and specific requirements of the medical device regulatory authorities participating in the MD-SAP program.

What is the meaning of ISO 13485 certified?

ISO certification is a seal of approval from a third party body that a company runs to one of the international standards developed and published by the International Organization for Standardization (ISO). ... ISO 13485 helps put your customers first.

Is ISO 13485 certification worth it?

ISO 13485 is important to designers, manufacturers, and distributors of medical devices. In addition, suppliers and service providers can enhance an organization's marketability as more and more manufacturers require certification in order to do business with a vendor.

MDSAP AUDIT:

The design and development of the MDSAP audit sequence allows a logical, focused and efficient conduct of an audit. The MDSAP audit sequence follows a process approach and has four primary processes - Management process, Measurement, Analysis and Improvement process, Design and Development process and a Production and Service Controls process with links to the supporting process for Purchasing.

The definition of each process includes a purpose and an outcome that are indicators of process performance. Each participating Regulatory Authority expects that risk management to be the foundation for the five processes that are the requirements of a quality management system for medical device organizations.

The MDSAP audit process has two additional supporting process-es: Device Marketing Authorization and Facility Registration and Medical Device Adverse Events and Advisory Notices Reporting. These processes are necessary to fulfill specific requirements of the participating MDSAP regulatory authorities.

Regulatory Requirements

Country	Regulatory	MDSAP
Australia	Conformity Assessment Procedures of the Australian Therapeutic Goods (Medical Devices) Regulations (TG(MD)R Sch3)	Page: 23
Brazil	The Brazilian Good Manufacturing Practices (RDC ANVISA 2013/16)	111
Canada	Medical Devices Regulations SOR/282-98 and specific requirements of the medical device regulatory authorities	213
Japan	The Japanese Ordinance on Standards for Manufacturing Control and Quality Control of Medical Devices and In Vitro Diagnostic Reagents (MHLW Ministerial Ordinance No. 169),	297
USA	FDA Quality System Regulation (21 CFR Part 820)	385

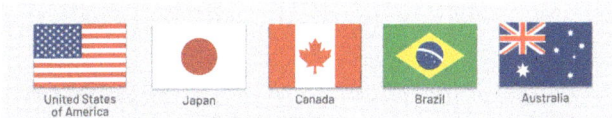

United States of America   Japan   Canada   Brazil   Australia

Definitions

ISO 13485 specifies requirements for a quality management system where an organization needs to demonstrate its ability to provide medical devices and related services that consistently meet customer and applicable regulatory requirements. Such organizations can be involved in one or more stages of the life-cycle, including design and development, production, storage and distribution, installation, or servicing of a medical device and design and development or provision of associated activities (e.g. technical support). ISO 13485 can also be used by suppliers or external parties that provide product, including quality management system-related services to such organizations.

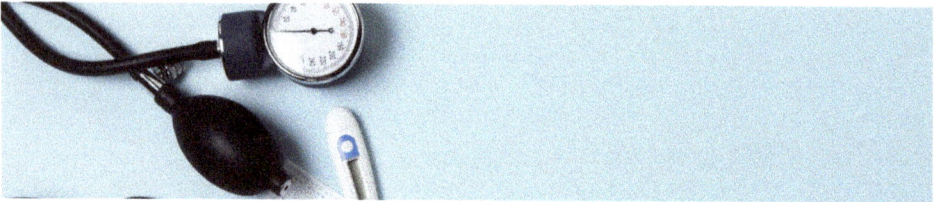

Scope of Certificate: The scope of the ISO certificate depends on how your Organization would like to have keeping in view of future. Some want to be specific by listing the products; some to be general covering the broad category of products. Here are some examples:

1. Design, development assemble, manufacture, distribute and service of life science instruments

2. Design, assemble/manufacture, sales & service of medical instruments used in cardiology including ECG Recorders, Bedside monitors

3. Design, development, manufacture, distribute and repair of medical device instruments intended to use in genetic analysis such as DNA Amplifiers, Genetic Analyzers, etc.

Distributer
Natural or legal person in the supply chain who, on his own behalf, furthers the availability of a medical device to the end user

Importer
natural or legal person in the supply chain who is the first in a supply chain to make a medical device,
manufactured in another country or jurisdiction, available in the country or jurisdiction where it is to
be marketed

Manufacturer
natural or legal person with responsibility for design and/or manufacture of a medical device with the
intention of making the medical device available for use, under his name; whether or not such a medical
device is designed and/or manufactured by that person himself or on his behalf by another person(s)

Device The term "device" is used throughout the MDSAP processes. For the purpose of applying the MDSAP processes, and to accommodate nuances in the regulatory systems of the participating Regulatory Authorities, the use of the term "device" is to refer to any product that is capable of functioning as a medical device, whether or not it is packaged, labeled, or sterilized.
Supplier: Organization or individual that enters into an agreement with the acquirer or integrator for the supply of a product or service.

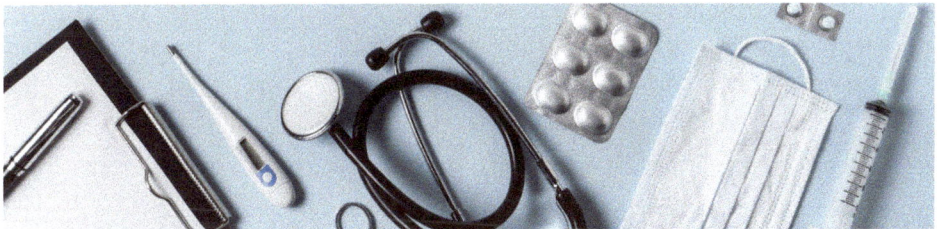

We can categorized the suppliers to:
- Critical Supplier
- Non-critical supplier

A purchased or otherwise obtained "product" or "service" is an outsourced product or service. In addition, a "supplier" is anyone that is independent from the medical device organization's quality management system. This includes a supplier that may be part of the same corporation as the medical device organization but operates under a separate quality management system from the audited medical device organization.

Critical Suppliers:

For the purposes of MDSAP, "critical suppliers" include, but are not limited to;

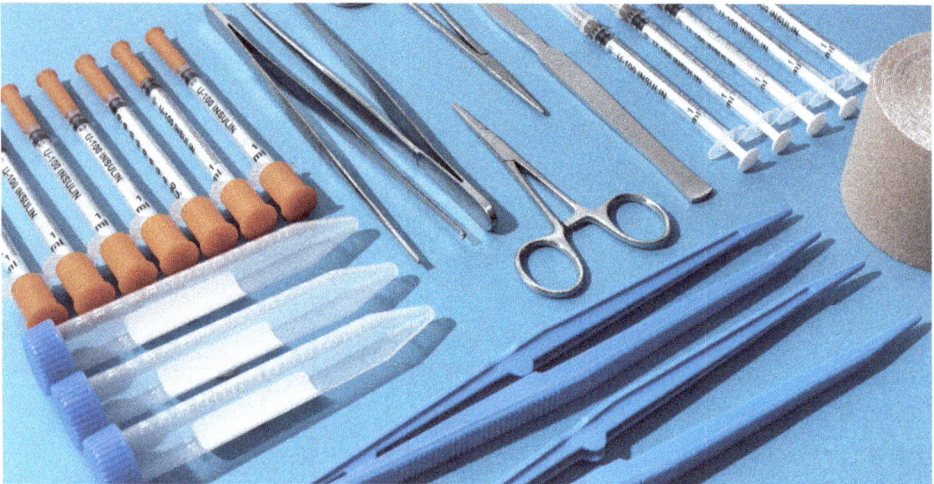

- Those entities that supply the organization with finished devices, i.e. a device, or accessory to any device, that is suitable for use or capable of functioning, whether or not it is packaged, labeled, or sterilized;
- Suppliers of products, including services, that impact design outputs that are essential for the proper functioning of the device; and
- Suppliers of products and services that require process validation.

Not all MDSAP participating regulatory authorities require, or make use of, certification documents that relate to a medical device organization's QMS. The terms "certification" and "recertification" appear within this volumes to maintain consistency with the terminology used within ISO/IEC 17021-1:2015 Conformity assessment – Requirements for bodies providing audit and certification of management systems.

MDSAP Audit

The Medical Device Single Audit Program is based on a three (3) year audit cycle. The Initial Audit, also referred to as the "Initial Certification Audit" is a complete audit of a medical device organization's quality management system (QMS) consisting of:

Stage 1 Audit (17021-1:2015 – Cl 9.3.1.2)

Stage 2 Audit (17021-1:2015 – Cl 9.3.1.3)

The initial Audit is followed by a partial Surveillance Audit (17021-1:2015 – Cl 9.6.2.2) in each of the following two (2) years and a complete Re-audit, also referred to as a "Recertification Audit" (17021-1:2015 – Cl 9.6.3.2) in the third (3rd) year. A recertification audit may also include a Stage 1 audit if there have been significant changes to the QMS that have not been otherwise adequately assessed.

Initial Certification Audit

Initial Certification audit consists of: Stage 1 & 2

Stage 1

Documentation review, evaluation of preparedness for Stage 2 audit, etc.

A Stage 1 audit shall be conducted in accordance with Clause 9.3.1.2 of ISO/IEC 17021-1:2015 and all applicable MDSAP Audit Process tasks and regulatory requirements.

From an MDSAP perspective, the primary purposes of a Stage 1 audit are (1) to determine if QMS documentation required by ISO 13485:2016 - Clauses 4.2.1 and other applicable MDSAP documentation requirements have been adequately defined, and documented; (2) to assess the medical device organization's preparedness for a Stage 2 audit; (3) to provide a focus for planning a Stage 2 audit; and, (4) to collect information regarding the scope of the quality management system and other aspects of the medical device organization.

Portions of a Stage 1 audit (e.g. documentation review) may be performed at a site other than the site(s) of the medical device organization seeking initial certification.

The outcome of the Stage 1 audit will assist the MDSAP recognized Auditing Organization in its determination of the readiness of the medical device organization to undergo a Stage 2 audit. The Au-

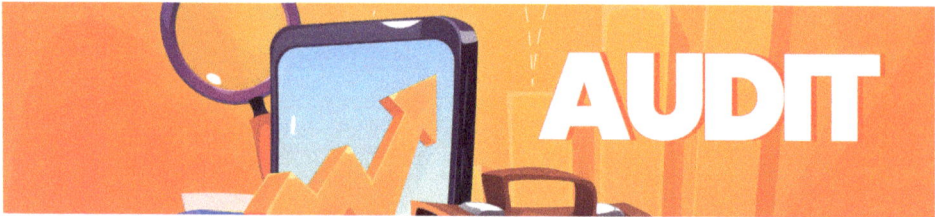

diting Organization shall determine how best to accomplish tasks of Stage 1 and Stage 2 with regards to off-site documentation and record review and on-site verifications. Hence portions of a Stage 1 audit (e.g. documentation review) may be performed at a site other than the site(s) of the medical device organization seeking initial certification. In practice it is intended that the Auditing Organization may combine elements of Stage 1 and Stage 2 to allow for a single on-site visit for the initial audit or re-audit of the medical device organization.

Stage 2

Evaluation of QMS Implementation and Effectiveness

A Stage 2 audit shall be conducted in accordance with Clause 9.3.1.3 of ISO/IEC 17021-1:2015 and using all applicable MDSAP Audit Process tasks.

The purpose of a Stage 2 audit is to determine if all applicable requirements of ISO 13485:2016 and the relevant regulatory requirements from participating regulatory authorities have been implemented. Stage 2 audit objectives shall specifically include an evaluation of:

- The effectiveness of the medical device organization's QMS incorporating the applicable regulatory requirements;
- Product/process related technologies (e.g. injection molding, sterilization);
- Adequate product technical documentation in relation to relevant regulatory requirements; and,
- The medical device organization's ability to comply with these requirements.

Surveillance Audits

(1st and 2nd Surveillance Audits):

A Surveillance Audit shall be conducted in accordance with Clause 9.6.2.2 of ISO/IEC 17021-1:2015 and clause 9.6.2 of IMDRF/MD-SAP WG/N3:2016 and using applicable MDSAP Audit Process tasks. The purpose of a series of surveillance audits is to assure that all applicable requirements of ISO 13485:2016 and the relevant regulatory requirements from participating regulatory authorities are audited during the cycle of a three year audit program for the medical device organization. Surveillance audit objectives during the audit cycle shall specifically include evaluation of:

- The effectiveness of the medical device organization's QMS incorporating the applicable regulatory requirements.
- The medical device organization's ability to comply with these requirements; and
- New or changed product/process related technologies; and,
- New or amended product technical documentation in relation to relevant regulatory requirements.

In addition, surveillance audits shall include a review of issues related to medical device safety and effectiveness since the last audit such as complaints, problem reports, vigilance reports, and recalls/field corrections/advisory notices.

Re-audit (Recertification Audits)

A Re-audit (Recertification Audit) shall be conducted in accordance with Clause 9.6.3 of ISO/IEC 17021-1:2015 and using all applicable MDSAP Audit Process tasks. The purpose of a re-audit is

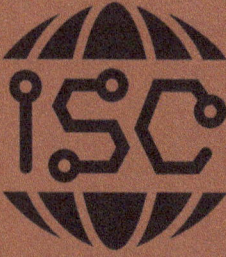

Sample Q

as a P

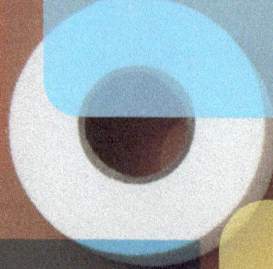

ISO 13

ME

Your Company
Quality Plan

Your Company
Organizational Chart

Your
Produc

Vision

Mi

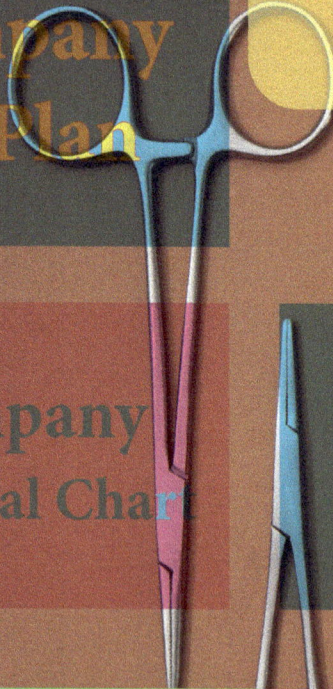

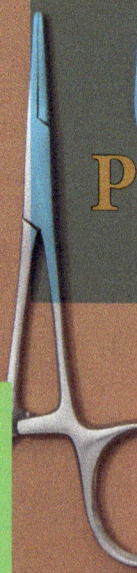

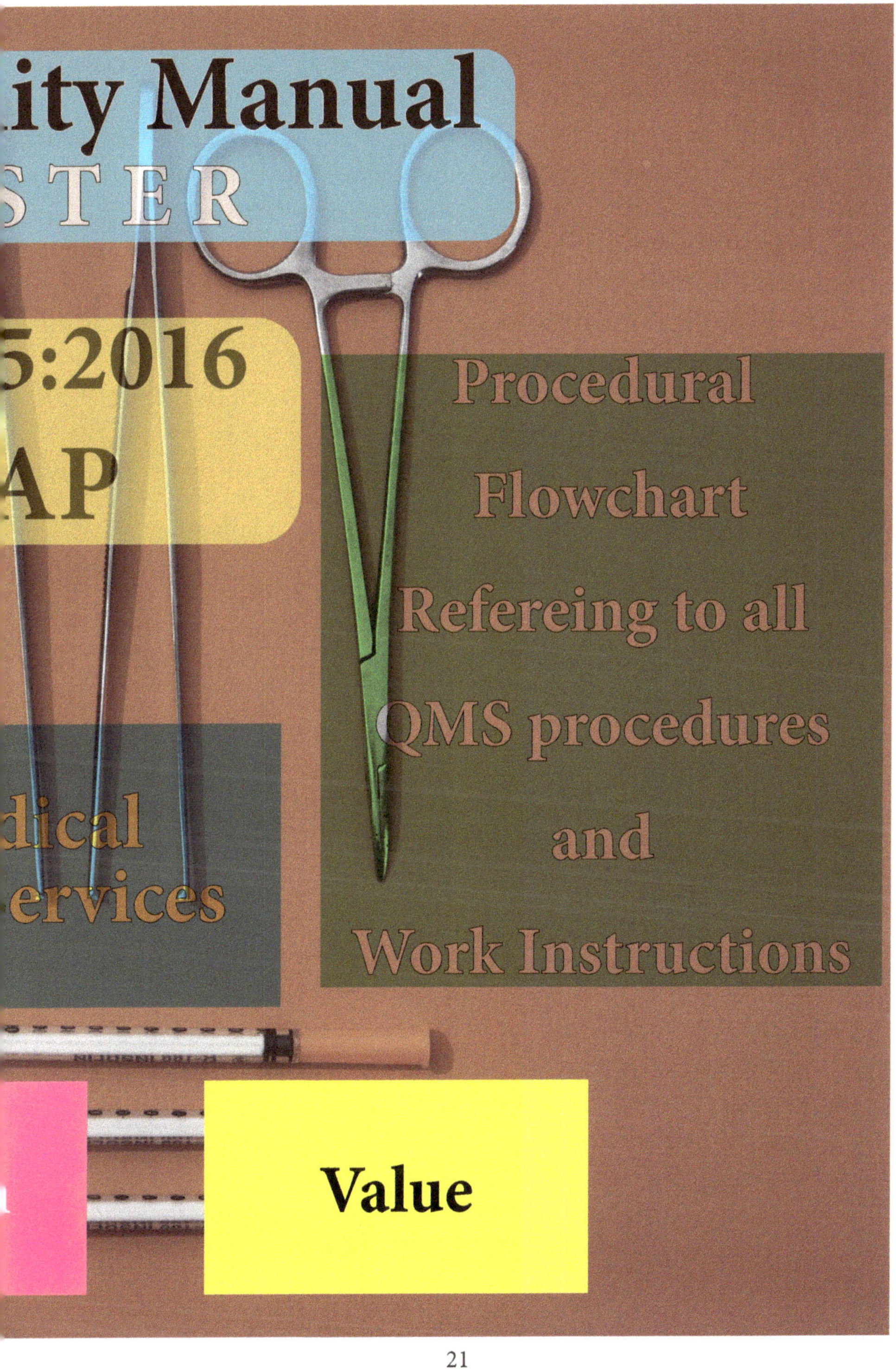

ity Manual
STER

5:2016
AP

dical
ervices

Procedural

Flowchart

Refereing to all

QMS procedures

and

Work Instructions

Value

to confirm the continued relevance, applicability and suitability of the medical device organization's QMS (as a whole), to satisfy all applicable requirements of ISO 13485:2016 and the relevant regulatory requirements from participating regulatory authorities, with respect to the scope of certification. Recertification audit objectives shall specifically include evaluation of:
- the effectiveness of the medical device organization's QMS incorporating the applicable regulatory requirements
- product/process related technologies (e.g. injection molding, sterilization)
- adequate product technical documentation in relation to relevant regulatory requirements
- the medical device organization's continued fulfillment of these requirements.

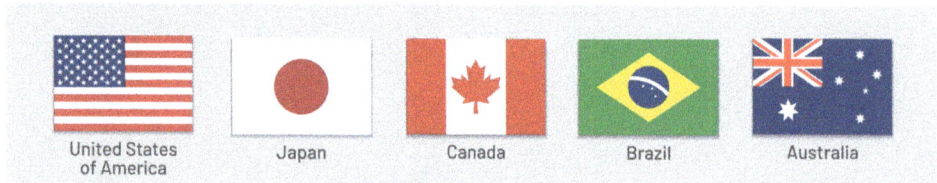

United States of America | Japan | Canada | Brazil | Australia

Audits Conducted by Regulatory Authorities

Audits may also be conducted by MDSAP participating regulatory authorities at any time and for a range of reasons including (1) "For Cause" due to information obtained by the regulatory authority, (2) as follow up to the findings of a previous audit, and (3) to confirm the effective implementation of MDSAP requirements by MDSAP recognized auditing organizations.

The purpose of audits conducted by regulatory authorities is to ensure appropriate oversight of a recognized MDSAP Auditing Organization's audit activities, as an alternative means of assessing medical device organizations that have been identified as undertaking high risk manufacturing processes and have not been adequately audited, where sufficient detail regarding audited processes has not been included in an audit report, or where there is a history of low compliance with QMS or regulatory requirements.

MDSAP
ISO 13485 Requirements

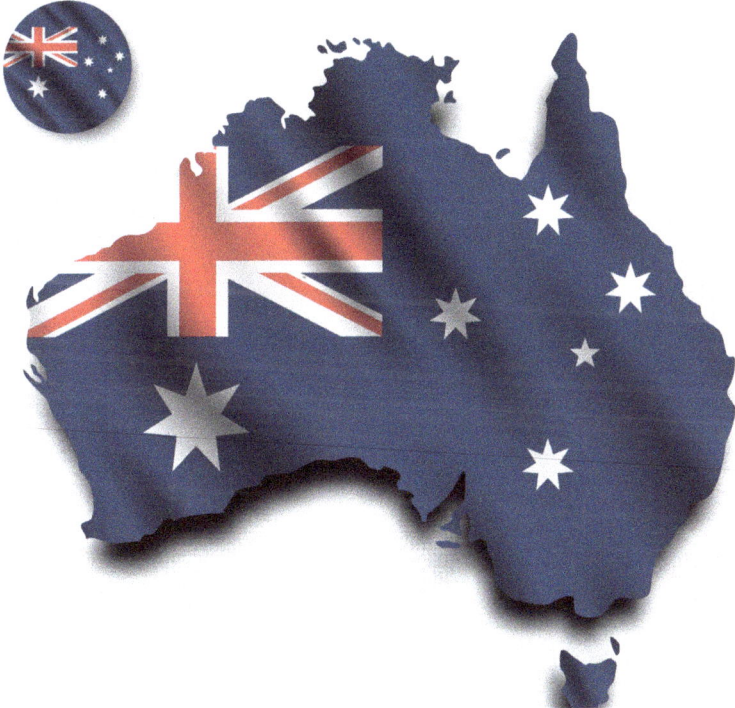

Management

The intent of the Management Process is to provide adequate resources for device design, manufacturing, quality assurance, distribution, installation, and servicing activities; to assure the quality management system is functioning properly and effectively; and to monitor the quality management system and make necessary adjustments. A quality management system that has been implemented effectively and is monitored to identify and address existing and potential problems is more likely to produce medical devices that function as intended.

The management representative is responsible for ensuring that the requirements of the quality management system have been effectively defined, documented, implemented, and maintained. Prior to the audit of a process, it may be helpful to interview the management representative (or designee) to obtain an overview of the process and a feel for management's knowledge and understanding of the process.

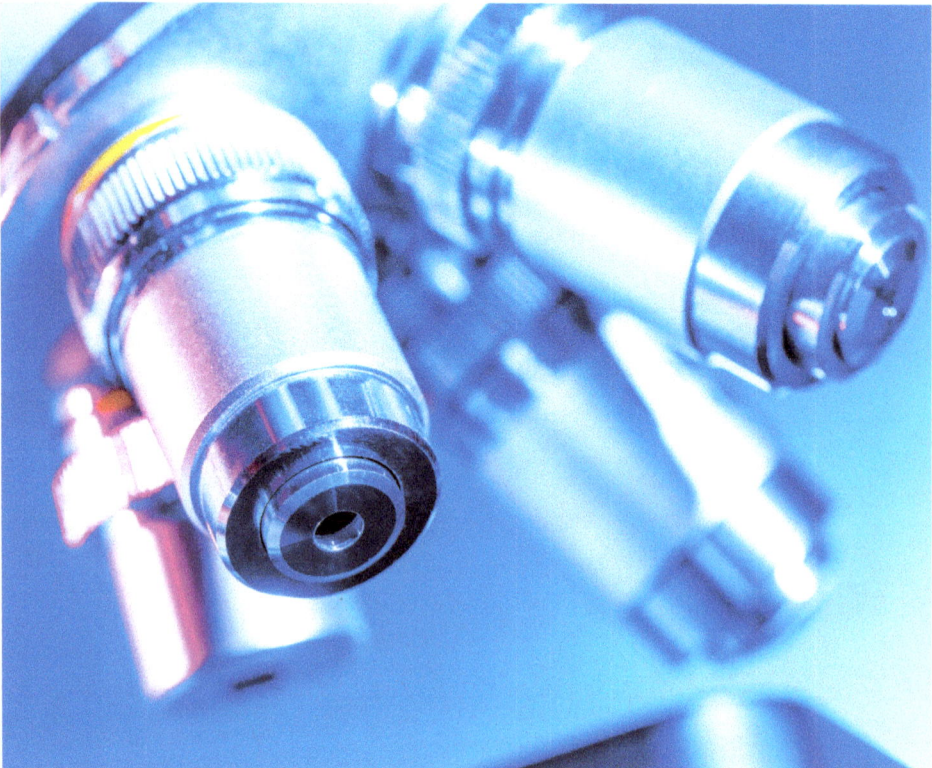

Clause and Regulation:
ISO 13485:2016: 4.1.1, 4.1.2, 4.1.3, 4.2.2, 4.1.4, 5.4.2;
TGA: TG(MD)R Sch3 P1 1.4(4);

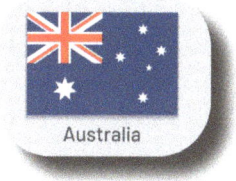

Australia

If an Australian Sponsor undertakes an activity that is preferred by the manufacturer, or required, to be under the control of the manufacturer, verify that the roles and responsibilities of the Australian Sponsor are documented in the manufacturer's quality management system and that the Sponsor is qualified and controlled as a supplier.

For example, but not limited to; a labeling activity to ensure that the name and address of the Australian Sponsor accompanies the device [TG(MD)R Reg 10.2], the installation of a device, or the servicing of a device.

Medical device market authorization, facility registration, and the submission of appropriate documentation to the TGA, are responsibilities of the Australian Sponsor. Australian manufacturers are also, by definition, Australian Sponsors.
For manufacturers located outside of Australia Confirm that the manufacturer is aware of the Australian Sponsor's entries in the Australian Register of Therapeutic Goods (ARTG).

Confirm that the manufacturer has a written agreement with the Australian Sponsor to ensure that information about the compliance of a device included in the ARTG, with the Essential Principles through the application of a relevant conformity assessment procedure, and information concerning adverse events, advisory notices and recalls is readily available to the Sponsor or the TGA.

The agreement must also require the Australian Sponsor to provide the manufacturer with any information in relation to the manufacturer's obligations under the conformity assessment procedures and any information in relation to whether the medical device complies with the Essential Principles.

Device Marketing Authorization and Facility Registration
The Device Marketing Authorization and Facility Registration process may be audited as a linkage from the Management process and/or the Design and Development process.

Therapeutic Goods Act

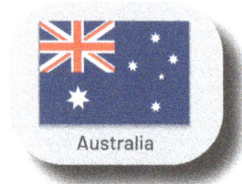
Australia

Manufacturer of a medical device is the person who is responsible for the design, production, packaging and labeling of the device before it is supplied under the person's name, whether or not it is the person, or another person acting on the person's behalf, who carries out those operations. A manufacturer of a medical device is also the person who, with a view to supplying the device under a person's name, does one or more of the following using ready made products: assembles, packages, processes, refurbishes, labels the device, or assigns a different intended purpose through the use of labels, instructions for use, advertising, or technical documentation (TG Act s41BG).

Australian importers (Sponsors) are required to include (register) medical devices from non-Australian Manufacturers in the Australian Register of Therapeutic Goods (ARTG). Sponsors are required to register the Manufacturers that they represent and to obtain a Client ID and Location ID for the manufacturer from the TGA.

To assist the Australian Sponsor, Manufacturers, who are supplying product to the Australian market and choose to participate in the MDSAP, must undertake the following to demonstrate that they have met the obligations on Manufacturers who wish to supply to Australia; Refer to following:

Therapeutic Goods Act
- Part 4-2 – Essential Principles and medical device standards
- Part 4-3 – Conformity Assessment Procedures
- Part 4-5 – Including medical devices in the Register
- Part 4-9 – Public Notification and recall of medical devices

Measurement, Analysis and Improvement

One of the most important activities in the quality management system is the identification of existing and potential causes of product and quality problems. Such causes must be identified so that appropriate and effective corrective or preventive actions can take place. These activities are carried out under the Measurement, Analysis and Improvement process.

Clause and Regulation

ISO: ISO 13485:2016: 4.2.1, 8.1, 8.2.1, 8.2.6, 8.5

TGA: TG(MD)R Sch3 P1 1.4(3)(a),(b), (5)(b) (iii), (f)

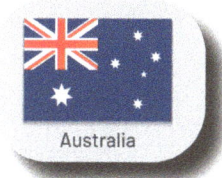

Australia

Confirm that when you plans to make a substantial change to a critical process (e.g. sterilization, processing materials of animal origin, processing materials of microbial or recombinant origin, or processes that incorporate a medicinal substance in a medical device), the manufacturer notifies the auditing organization who will determine if an assessment of the change is required before implementation.

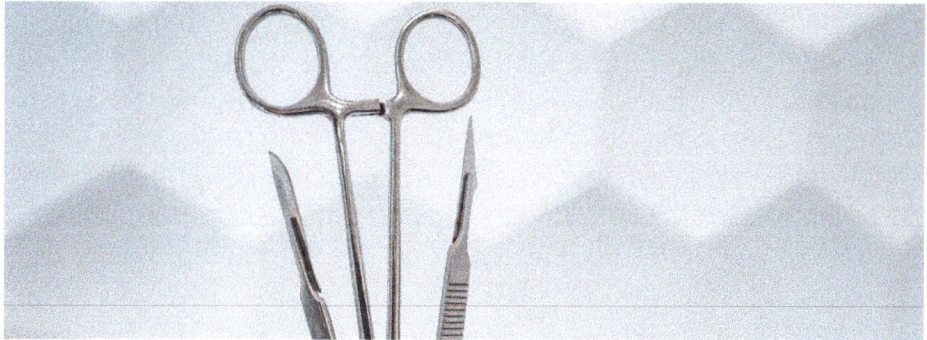

Verify that the organization has procedures for a post-marketing system that includes a systematic review of post-production experience (e.g. from; expert user groups, customer surveys, customer complaints and warranty claims, service and repair information, literature reviews, post-production clinical trials, user feedback other than complaints, device tracking and registration schemes, user reactions during training, adverse event reports). Investigation should take place in a timely manner to ensure that reporting time frames for adverse events or advisory notices may be met.

Medical Device Adverse Events and Advisory Notices Reporting
The Medical Device Adverse Events and Advisory Notices Reporting
process may be audited as a linkage from the Measurement, Analysis
and Improvement process.

Clause and Regulation
ISO: ISO 13485:2016: 4.2.1, 7.2.3, 8.2.2, 8.2.3
TGA: TG(MD)R Sch3 P1 1.4(3)(c)(i)

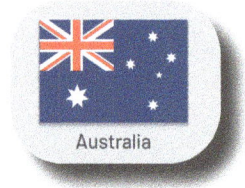

Australia

You are required to implement a post-marketing system that includes provisions for adverse event reporting – e.g. Therapeutic Goods (Medical Devices) Regulations 2002 Schedule 3 Part 1
Clause 1.4(3)(c)(i).
In view of the written agreement between Manufacturers and the
Australian Sponsor [TG Act 41FD], events must be reported by the
Manufacturer to the TGA, or to the Sponsor, in a timely manner to
ensure that a Sponsor can meet their reporting obligations under
the Therapeutic Goods (Medical Devices) Regulation 5.7:

- Verify that the Manufacturer or other person becoming aware
  of an event that represents a serious threat to public health
  provides information as soon as practicable. The Sponsor is to
  report the event within 48 hours.
- Verify that the Manufacturer or other person becoming aware
  of an event that led to the death or serious deterioration in the
  state of health of a patient, a user, or other person provides
  information as soon as practicable. The Sponsor is to report the
  event within 10 days.
- Verify that the manufacturer or other person becoming aware of
  an event that the recurrence of which might lead to the death or
  serious deterioration in the state of health of a patient, a user, or
  other person provides information as soon as practicable. The
  Sponsor is to report the event within 30 days.

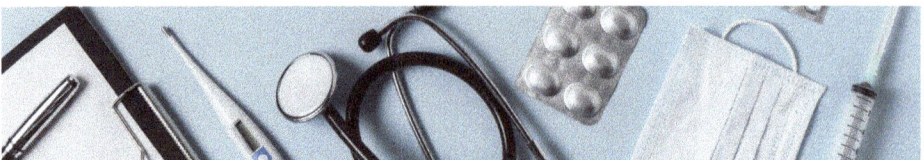

It is a condition on Australian Sponsors of Class AIMD, Class III and Implantable Class IIb devices that they provide three consecutive annual reports to the TGA following inclusion of the device in the ARTG. Annual reports are due 1 October each year. Reports should be for the period 1 July to 30 June. The report is to include:
- ARTG no.
- Product name
- Model no(s)
- Number supplied in Australia

Number supplied worldwide (Numbers should include devices that are the same but supplied under a different name in another jurisdiction)
- Number of complaints in Australia
- Number of complaints worldwide
- Number of adverse events and incident rates in Australia (Rate= No. of events/ No. Supplied x 100 = Rate%)
- Number of adverse events and incident rates world wide
- A list of the more common complaints and all of the adverse events
- Device Incident Report (DIR) number of those adverse events reported to the TGA
- Regulatory/corrective action/notification by Manufacturer

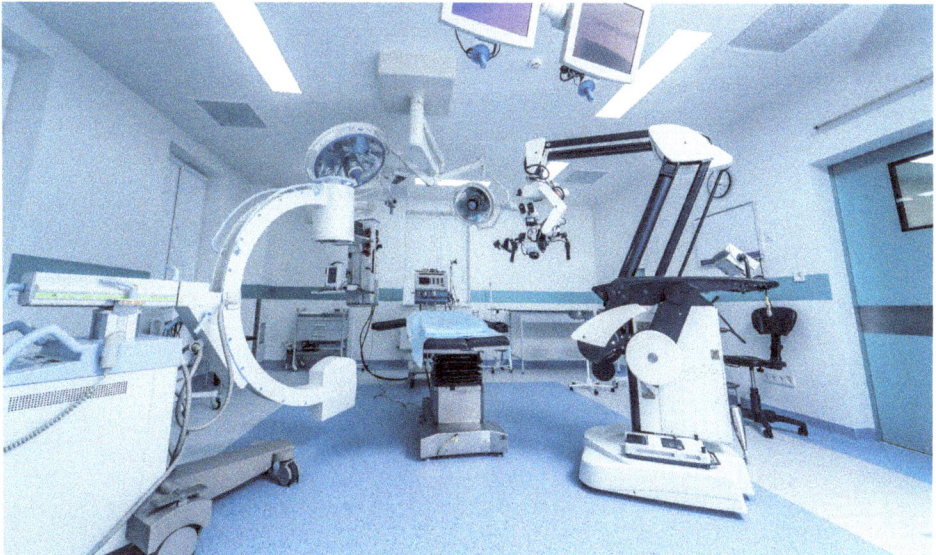

Canada

Class IV
Class III
Class II
Class I

USA

Class III
Class II
Class I

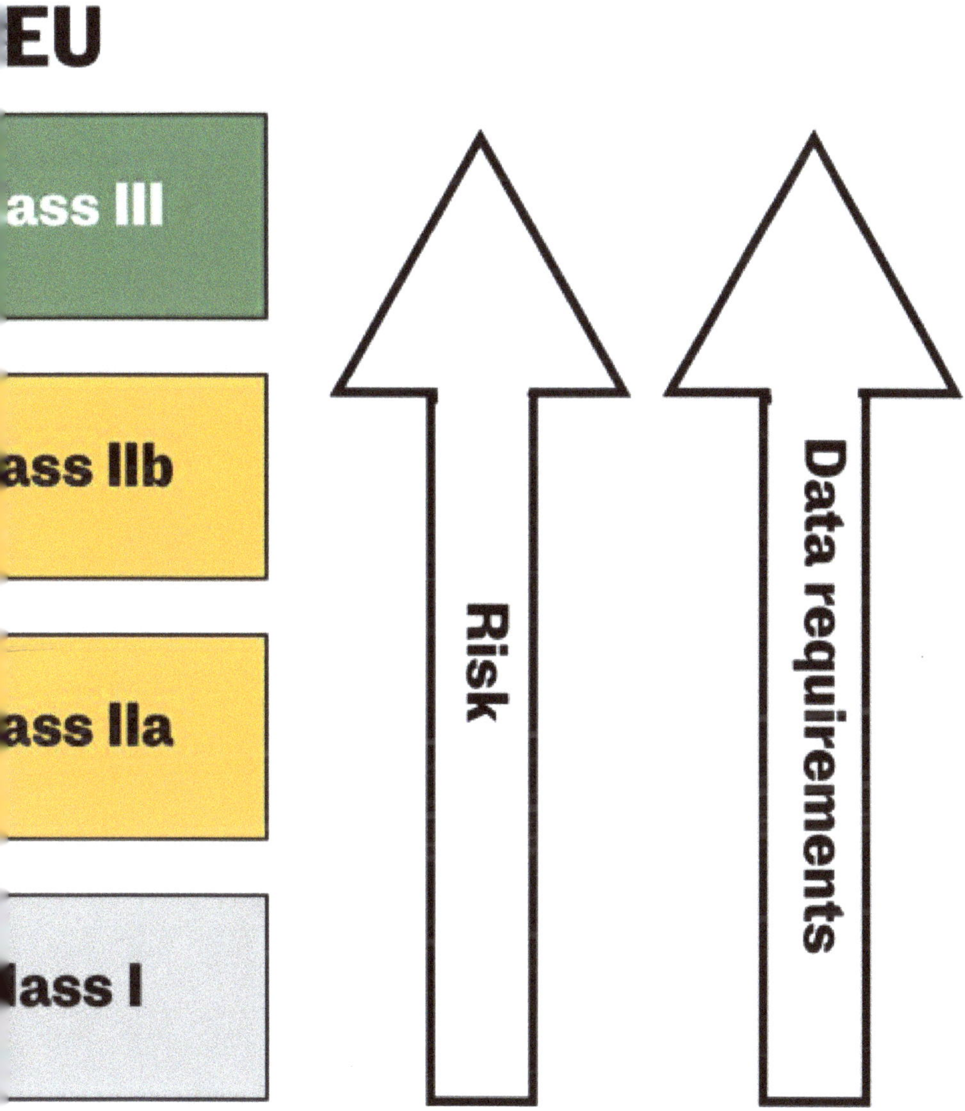

EU

Class III

Class IIb

Class IIa

Class I

Risk

Data requirements

Design and Development

The purpose of the Design and Development process is to control the design of a medical device and to assure that the device meets user needs, intended use, and its specified requirements. Attention to design and development planning, identifying design inputs, developing design outputs, verifying that design outputs meet design inputs, validating the design, controlling design changes, reviewing design results, transferring the design to production, and compiling the appropriate records will help a medical device organization assure that resulting designs will meet user needs, intended uses, and requirements. Review of the Design and Development process will also provide an opportunity to evaluate how the medical device organization has utilized risk management activities to ensure design inputs are comprehensive and meet user needs, to confirm that risk control measures that were planned have been implemented in the design, and to verify that risk control measures are effective in controlling or reducing risk.

Clause and Regulation
ISO: ISO 13485:2016: 4.1.1, 4.2.1, 7.1, 7.3.10
TGA: TG(MD)R Division 3.2

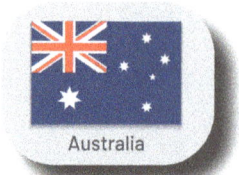

Australia

When you applies TG(MD)R Division 3.2 and selects the Full Quality Assurance conformity assessment procedures [TG(MR)R Schedule 3, Part1, (excluding or including clause 1.6)], quality management system procedures for design and development must be available.

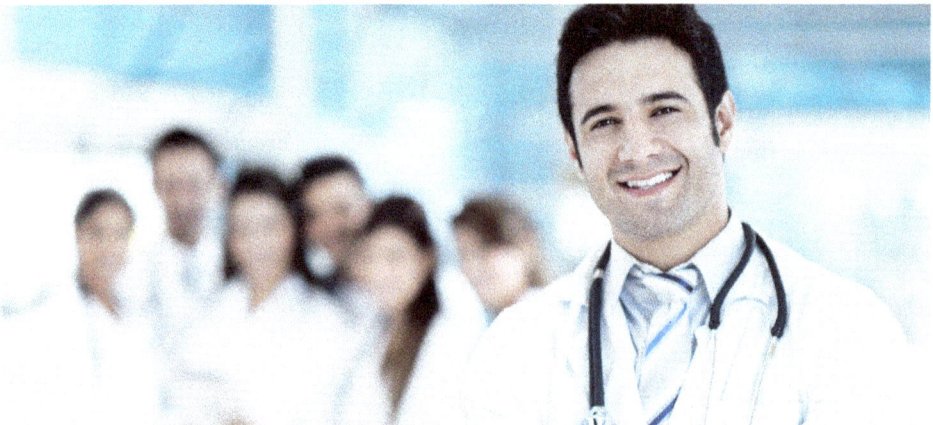

Production and Service Controls

The purpose of the Production and Service Controls process is to manufacture products that meet specifications. Developing processes that are adequate to produce devices that meet specifications, validating (or fully verifying the results of) those processes, and monitoring and controlling those processes are all steps that help assure the result will be devices that meet specified requirements. After completing the audit of the medical device organization's Production and Service Controls process, the audit team will return to the Management process to make a final decision of whether top management ensures that an adequate and effective quality management system has been established and maintained at the medical device organization.

Clause and Regulation
ISO: ISO 13485:2016: 7.1, 7.2.1, 7.5.1
TGA: TG(MD)R Sch 1 P1 2, Sch3 P1 Cl1.4(4), Sch3 P1 Cl1.4(5)(d)&(e)

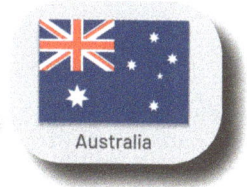

Australia

Confirm that methods of validation have regard to the generally acknowledged state of the art (e.g. current Medical Device Standard Orders - MDSO, ISO/IEC Standards, BP, EP, USP etc.)
Verify that methods of sterilization validation have regard to the generally acknowledged state of the art (e.g. current Australian Medical Device Standard Orders - MDSO, ISO 11135, ISO 11137)

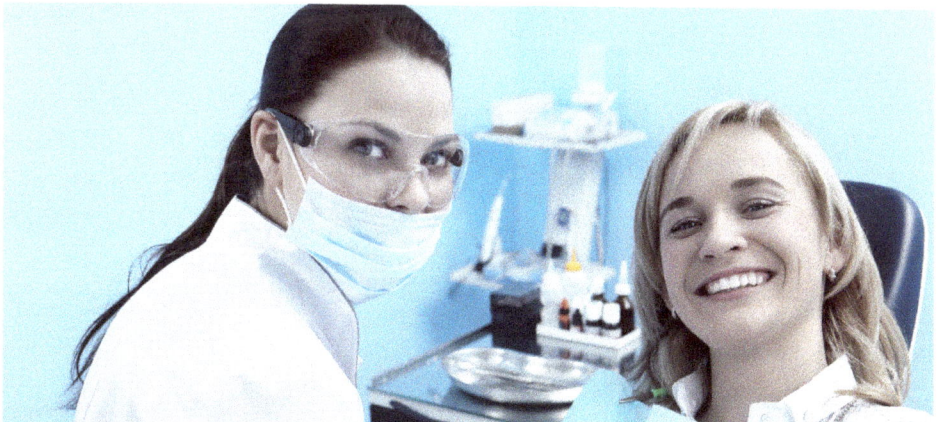

Reviewing a validation
During review of a validation study, determine when applicable whether:

- The instruments used to generate the data were properly calibrated and maintained
- Predetermined product and process specifications were established
- Sampling plans used to collect test samples are based on a statistically valid rationale
- Data demonstrates predetermined specifications were met consistently
- Process tolerance limits were challenged
- Process equipment was properly installed, adjusted, and maintained
- Process monitoring instruments were properly calibrated and maintained
- Changes to the validated process were appropriately challenged (if applicable)
- Process operators were appropriately qualified.

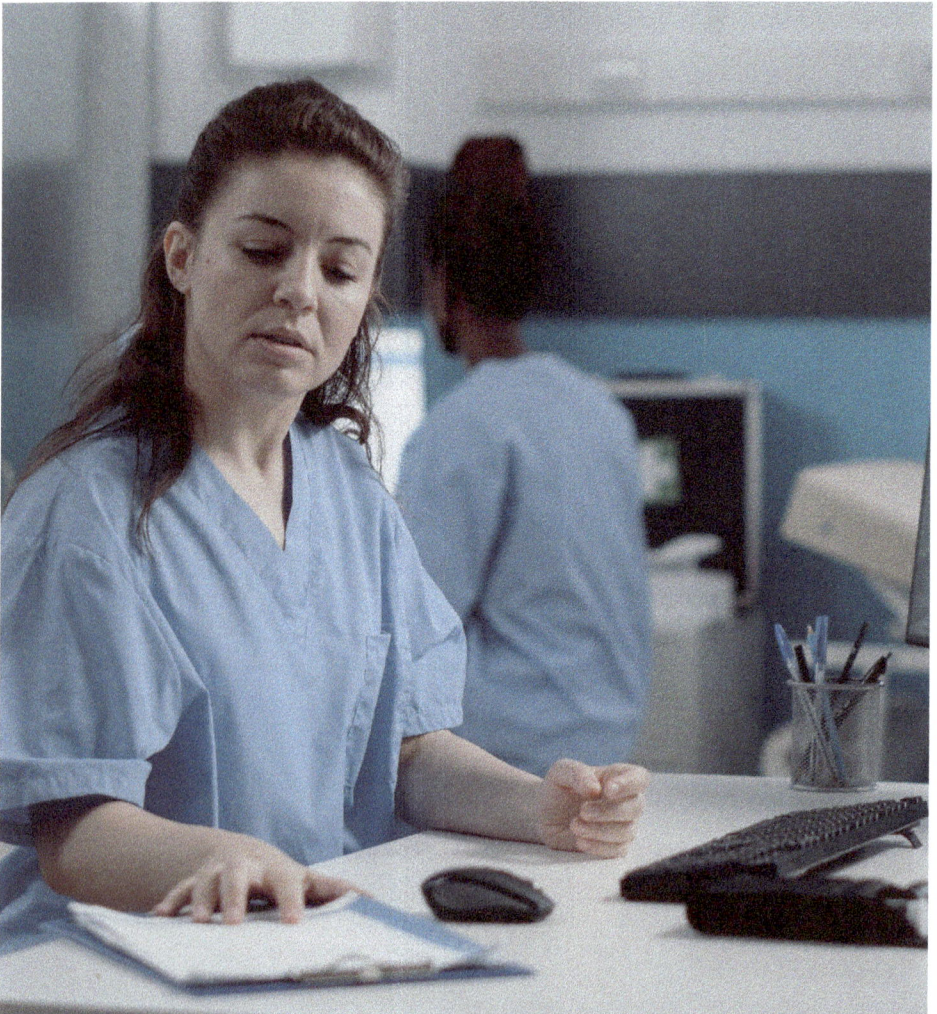

Purchasing

The intent of the Purchasing process is to ensure that purchased, sub-contracted, or otherwise received products and services conform to specified requirements. The medical device organization is expected to establish and maintain documented controls for planning and performing purchasing activities. The controls necessary depend on the effect of the product on the quality, safety, and effectiveness of the finished device. Effective purchasing processes incorporate purchasing requirements and specifications, the selection of acceptable suppliers based on the capability of the suppliers to provide acceptable product, the performance of necessary acceptance activities, and maintenance of the required quality records.

The management representative is responsible for ensuring that the requirements of the quality management system have been effectively defined, documented, implemented, and maintained. Prior to the audit of a process, it may be helpful to interview the management representative to obtain an overview of the process and a feel for management's knowledge and understanding of the process.

Clause and Regulation
ISO: ISO: ISO 13485:2016: 4.1.2, 4.1.3, 4.1.5, 7.1, 7.4.1, 7.4.2, 7.4.3
TGA: TG(MD)R Sch1 P1 2, Sch3 P1 Cl1.4(5)(d)(ii)

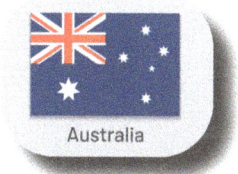

Australia

Planning

In planning product realization, the medical device organization must determine as appropriate the quality objectives and requirements for the purchased products, the processes, documents, and resources specific to the purchased products, the criteria for purchased product acceptance, and the required verification, monitoring, inspection, and test activities specific to the purchased products. Planning of product realization often begins in the design and development of the product, including the translation of the design into production specifications. The translation of the design into production specifications includes the establishment of specified requirements for purchased product.

Quality objectives

Quality objectives are typically expressed as a measurable target or goal. The planning of product realization should include consideration of how the purchased product, the criteria for purchased product acceptance, and the required verification, monitoring, inspection, and test activities specific to the purchased product will achieve the quality objectives.

- Some examples of QOB include:
- Number of complaints -v- number of parts shipped
- On-time delivery %
- Supplier parts rejected
- Comparison of internal audit findings -v- external audit findings
- Achieving a certain accuracy if you're developing product - based software
- Annual Post-market surveillance
- Auditing our system for regulatory compliance

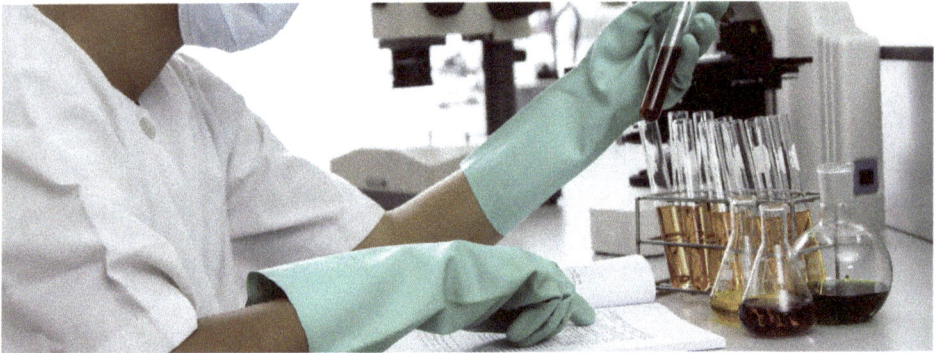

Some managers believe that the reward for hard work should be a paycheck. That's sort of like telling your children that they get to eat for doing something you're proud of. Employees are not children, but you are responsible for developing them into more valuable employees so that they can be promoted. If there is no incentive, your team will not be engaged. Therefore, pick a reward that is proportional to the bottom-line impact. Five percent of the bottom-line impact is what I like to target, but you would be amazed at how effective a few small rewards at each milestone can be. If you have trouble getting management approval for rewards, remind your boss of the bottom-line impact and link the rewards closely to the impact.

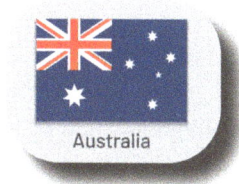

Australia

MDSAP
Audit Checklist

		REQUIREMENTS
		4 Quality management system
		4.1 General requirements
		Has the organization:
		a) identified the processes needed for the quality management system and their application throughout the organization (see 1.2)?
		b) determined the sequence and interaction of these processes?
		c) determined criteria and methods needed to ensure that both the operation and control of these processes are effective?
		d) ensured the availability of resources and information necessary to support the operation and monitoring of their processes?
		e) monitored, measured, and analyzed these processes
		f) implemented actions necessary to achieve planned results and maintain the effectiveness of these processes?
		Does the organization manage these processes in accordance with the requirements of this International Standard?
		Where an organization chooses to outsource any process that affects product conformity with requirements, does the organization ensure control over such processes?
		Is the control of such outsourced processes identified within the quality management system? (see 8.5.1)
	Australia	If an Australian Sponsor undertakes an activity that is preferred by the manufacturer, or required, to be under the control of the manufacturer, verify that the roles and responsibilities of the Australian Sponsor are documented in the manufacturer's quality management system and that the Sponsor is qualified and controlled as a supplier.

Doc. Reference	Adequate?	Stage I (clauses marked *)	Stage II
	Y/N	Initial›s	Initial›s

	REQUIREMENTS

4.2.1 General	
	Does the quality management system documentation include:
	a) documented statements of a quality policy and quality objectives?
	b) a quality manual?
	c) documented procedures required by this international standard?
	d) documents needed by the organization to ensure the effective planning, operation and control of its processes?
	e) records required by this International Standard (see 4.2.4)?
	f) any other documentation specified by national or regional regulations?
	Has the organization established and maintained a file for each type or model of medical device either containing or identifying documents defining product specifications and quality system requirements (see 4.2.3)?
	Do these documents define the complete manufacturing process and, if applicable, installation and servicing?

Doc. Reference	Adequate?	Stage I (clauses marked *)	Stage II

	REQUIREMENTS
Australia	Verify that the manufacturer prepares and maintains complete and current objective evidence that demonstrates compliance with the Essential Principles of Safety and Performance [TG(MD)R Sch3 P5)1.4 1)(c) & 1.9].
	Verify that devices to be sold in Australia have labeling and instructions for use that comply with the Essential Principles for information that is to be provided with a device [TG(MD)R Sch1 P13 2]. When the Therapeutic Goods (Medical Devices) Regulations 2002 does not require a manufacturer to apply design and development controls for the Class of the medical device (Class IIa, Class I Measuring, Class I Sterile), the manufacturer shall prepare and maintain complete and current objective evidence that demonstrates compliance with the Essential Principles of Safety and Performance [see TG(MD)R Sch3 P6.4 6 - Required Technical Documentation].
4.2.2 Quality manual	
	Has the organization established and maintained a quality manual that includes:
	a) the scope of the quality management system, including details of and justification for any exclusion and/or non-application (see 1.2)?
	b) the documented procedures established for the quality management system, or reference to them?
	c) a description of the interaction between the processes of the quality management system?
	Does the quality manual outline the structure of the documentation used in the quality management system?

Doc. Reference	Adequate?	Stage I (clauses marked *)	Stage II

	REQUIREMENTS
Australia	For manufacturers located outside of Australia: Confirm that the manufacturer is aware of the Australian Sponsor's entries in the Australian Register of Therapeutic Goods (ARTG) Confirm that the manufacturer has a written agreement with the Australian Sponsor to ensure that information about the compliance of a device included in the ARTG, with the Essential Principles through the application of a relevant conformity assessment procedure, and information concerning adverse events, advisory notices and recalls is readily available to the Sponsor or the TGA. The agreement must also require the Australian Sponsor to provide the manufacturer with any information in relation to the manufacturer's obligations under the conformity assessment procedures and any information in relation to whether the medical device complies with the Essential Principles [TG Act s41FD, s41FN(3)(e), TG(MD)R Sch3 P1 Cl3)1.4), Cl1.7].
EU	Are the applicable sections of the Medical Device Directive (MDD) included in the specified requirements throughout the documented quality system? Interpretation: A statement only indicating compliance/conformity with the relevant international or EU regulatory requirements is not acceptable.
4.2.3 Control of documents	
	Are documents required by the quality management system controlled?

Doc. Reference	Adequate?	Stage I (clauses marked *)	Stage II

	REQUIREMENTS
	Is a documented procedure established to define the controls needed:
	a) To review and approve documents for adequacy prior to issue?
	b) To review and update as necessary and re-approve documents?
	c) To ensure that changes and the current revision status of documents are identified?
	d) To ensure that relevant versions of applicable documents are available at points of use?
	e) To ensure the documents remain legible and readily identifiable?
	f) To ensure that documents of external origin are identified and their distribution controlled?
	g) To prevent the unintended use of obsolete documents and to apply suitable identification to them if they are retained for any purpose?
	Does the organization ensure that changes to documents are reviewed and approved either by the original approving function or another designated function which has access to pertinent background information upon which to base its decisions?
	Does the organization define the period for which at least one copy of obsolete controlled documents shall be retained?
	Does this period ensure that documents to which medical devices have been manufactured and tested are available for at least the lifetime of the medical device as defined by the organization, but not less than the retention period of any resulting record (see 4.2.4), or as specified by relevant regulatory requirements?

Doc. Reference	Adequate?	Stage I (clauses marked *)	Stage II

	REQUIREMENTS
Australia	Confirm that Quality Management System documentation and records in relation to a device are retained by the manufacturer for at least 5 years [TG(MD)R Sch3 P1.9 1].
4.2.4 Control of quality records	
	Are records established and maintained to provide evidence of conformity to requirements and of the effective operation of the quality management system?
	Do records remain legible, readily identifiable and retrievable?
	Has a documented procedure been established to define the controls needed for the identification, storage, protection, retrieval, retention time and disposition of records?
	Does the organization retain the records for a period of time at least equivalent to the lifetime of the medical device as defined by the organization, but not less than two years from the date of product release by the organization or as specified by relevant regulatory requirements?
EU	Has the manufacturer retained for a period ending at least five years after the last product has been manufactured, the records listed in Annex II, 6.1 or Annex V, 5.1 or Annex VI, 5.1 (whichever applies)
5 Management responsibility	
5.1 Management commitment	

Doc. Reference	Adequate?	Stage I (clauses marked *)	Stage II

	REQUIREMENTS
	Has top management provided evidence of its commitment to the development and implementation of the quality management system and maintaining its effectiveness by:
	a) Communicating to the organization the importance of meeting customer as well as statutory and regulatory requirements?
	b) Establishing the quality policy?
	c) Ensuring that quality objectives are established?
	d) Conducting management reviews?
	e) Ensuring the availability of resources?
5.2 Customer focus	
	Does top management ensure that customer requirements are determined and met (see 7.2.1 and 8.2.1)?
5.3 Quality policy	
	Does top management ensure that the quality policy
	a) Is appropriate to the purpose of the organization?
	b) Includes a commitment to comply with requirements and to maintain the effectiveness of the quality management system?
	c) Provides a framework for establishing and reviewing quality objectives?
	d) Is communicated and understood within the organization?
	e) Is reviewed for continuing suitability?
5.4 Planning	
5.4.1 Quality objectives	
	Does top management ensure that quality objectives, including those needed to meet requirements for product (see 7.1a), are established at relevant functions and levels within the organization?
	Are quality objectives measurable?

Doc. Reference	Adequate?	Stage I (clauses marked *)	Stage II

	REQUIREMENTS	
	Are quality objectives consistent with the quality policy?	
5.4.2 Quality management system planning		
	Has top management ensured that:	
	a) The planning of the quality management system is carried out in order to meet the requirements given in 4.1, as well as the quality objectives?	
	b) The integrity of the quality management system is maintained when changes to the quality management system are planned and implemented?	
5.5 Responsibility, authority and communication		
5.5.1 Responsibility and authority		
	Has top management ensured that responsibilities and authorities were defined, documented and communicated within the organization?	
	Has top management established the interrelation of all personnel who manage, perform and verify work affecting quality, and ensured the independence and authority necessary to perform these tasks?	
5.5.2 Management representative		
	Has top management appointed a member of management who, irrespective of other responsibilities, has responsibility and authority that includes:	
	a) Ensuring that processes needed for the quality management system are established, implemented, and maintained?	
	b) Reporting to top management on the performance of the quality management system and any need for improvement (see 8.5)?	
	c) Ensuring the promotion of awareness of regulatory and customer requirements throughout the organization?	
5.5.3 Internal communication		

Doc. Reference	Adequate?	Stage I (clauses marked *)	Stage II

	REQUIREMENTS
	Has top management ensured that appropriate communication processes have been established within the organization and that communication takes place regarding the effectiveness of the quality management system?
5.6 Management review	
5.6.1 General	
	Does top management review the organization's quality management system, at planned intervals, to ensure its continuing suitability, adequacy and effectiveness?
	Does this review include assessing opportunities for improvement and the need for changes to the quality management system, including the quality policy and quality objectives?
	Are records from management reviews maintained (see 4.2.4)?
5.6.2 Review input	
	Does the input to management review include information on:
	a) Results of audits?
	b) Customer feedback?
	c) Process performance and product conformity?
	d) Status of preventive and corrective actions?
	e) Follow-up actions from previous management reviews?
	f) Changes that could affect the quality management system?
	g) Recommendations for improvement?
	h) New or revised regulatory requirements?

Doc. Reference	Adequate?	Stage I (clauses marked *)	Stage II

	REQUIREMENTS
	5.6.3 Review output
	Does output from the management review include any decisions and actions related to:
	a) Improvements needed to maintain the effectiveness of the quality management system and its processes?
	b) Improvement of product related to customer requirements?
	c) Resource needs?
	6 Resource management
	6.1 Provision of resources
	Does the organization determine and provide the resources needed:
	a) To implement the quality management system and to maintain its effectiveness?
	b) To meet regulatory and customer requirements?
	6.2 Human resources
	6.2.1 General
	Are personnel performing work affecting product quality competent on the basis of appropriate education, training, skills and experience?
	6.2.2 Competence, awareness and training

Doc. Reference	Adequate?	Stage I (clauses marked *)	Stage II

	REQUIREMENTS
	Does the organization:
	a) determine the necessary competence for personnel performing work affecting product quality?
	b) Provide training or take other actions to satisfy these needs?
	c) Evaluate the effectiveness of actions taken?
	d) Ensure that its personnel are aware of the relevance and importance of their activities and how they contribute to the achievement of the quality objectives?
	e) Maintain appropriate records of education, training, skills and experience (see 4.2.4)?
6.3 Infrastructure	
	Does the organization determine, provide and maintain the infrastructure needed to achieve conformity to product requirements?
	Infrastructure includes, as applicable:
	a) Buildings, workspace and associated utilities
	b) Process equipment, both hardware and software
	c) Supporting services such as transport or communication
	Does the organization establish documented requirements for maintenance activities, including their frequency, when such activities or lack thereof can affect product quality?
	Are records of such maintenance maintained (see 4.2.4)?
	Has the organization determined and does it manage the work environment needed to achieve conformity to product requirements?
	a) Has the organization established documented requirements for health, cleanliness and clothing of personnel if contact between such personnel and the product or work environment could adversely affect the quality of the product (see 7.5.1.2.1)?

Doc. Reference	Adequate?	Stage I (clauses marked *)	Stage II

	REQUIREMENTS
	b) If work environment conditions can have an adverse effect on product quality, has organization established documented requirements for the work environment conditions and documented procedures or work instructions to monitor and control these work environment conditions (see 7.5.1.2.1)?
	c) Does the organization ensure that all personnel who are required to work temporarily under special environmental conditions within the work environment are appropriately trained or supervised by a trained person [see 6.2.2 b)]?
	d) If appropriate, are special arrangements established and documented for the control of contaminated or potentially contaminated product in order to prevent contamination of other product, the work environment or personnel (see 7.5.3.1)?
7 Product realization	
7.1 Planning of product realization	
	Has the organization planned and developed the processes needed for product realization?
	Is the planning of product realization consistent with the requirements of the other processes of the quality management system (see 4.1)?

Doc. Reference	Adequate?	Stage I (clauses marked *)	Stage II

	REQUIREMENTS
	In planning product realization, has the organization determined the following, as appropriate:
	a) Quality objectives and requirements for products?
	b) The need to establish processes, documents, and provide resources specific to the product?
	c) Required verification, validation, monitoring, inspection and test activities specific to the product and the criteria for product acceptance?
	d) Records needed to provide evidence that the realization processes and resulting product meet requirements (see 4.2.4)?
	Is the output of this planning in a form suitable for the organization's method of operations?
	Does the organization establish documented requirements for risk management throughout product realization and are records arising from risk management maintained (see 4.2.4)?
Australia	Confirm that when a manufacturer plans to make a substantial change to a critical process (e.g. sterilization, processing materials of animal origin, processing materials of microbial or recombinant origin, or processes that incorporate a medicinal substance in a medical device), the manufacturer notifies the auditing organization who will determine if an assessment of the change is required before implementation [TG(MD)R Sch3 P2)1.5 1)].
EU	Does the supplier evaluate the need for risk analysis throughout the design process and maintain records of any risk analysis performed? (MDD Annex 1)

Doc. Reference	Adequate?	Stage I (clauses marked *)	Stage II

	REQUIREMENTS

7.2.1 Determination of requirements related to the product	
	Has the organization determined:
	a) Requirements specified by the customer, including the requirements for delivery and post-delivery activities?
	b) Requirements not stated by the customer but necessary for specified or intended use, where known?
	c) Statutory and regulatory requirements related to the product?
	d) Any additional requirements determined by the organization?

Doc. Reference	Adequate?	Stage I (clauses marked *)	Stage II

	REQUIREMENTS

Australia	Verify that the Australian importers (Sponsors) has included (register) medical devices from non-Australian manufacturers in the Australian Register of Therapeutic Goods (ARTG).
	verifyy that the non-Australian manufacturers has assisted the Australian Sponsor by undertaking the following tasks to demonstrate that they have met the obligations on manufacturers who wish to supply to Australia;
	  - Classify the device using the Australian classification rules
	  - Identify an Australian conformity assessment procedure that is to be applied in accordance with the classification of the device
	  - Obtain 3rd party assessment of their QMS and the device in accordance with the selected conformityvassessment procedure or an equivalent EU MDD, AIMD or IVDD procedure
	  - Prepare an Australian Declaration of Conformity in accordance with the requirements of the Conformity Assessment Procedure that has been applied [TG(MD)R Sch 3 P1 Cl1.8].
	     o If requested to do so by an authorized person, produce to the person such documents relatingvto devices of the kind included in the Register as the person requires and allow the person tovcopy the documents
	   o That the manufacturer will comply with any conditions imposed on the manufacture of devices
	   o That the Sponsor provide the manufacturer with information in relation to the manufacturer's obligations under a conformity assessment procedure and information in relation to whether the devices comply with the Essential Principles [TG Act 41FN(3)(e)].

Doc. Reference	Adequate?	Stage I (clauses marked *)	Stage II

	REQUIREMENTS
EU	Vefiy that manufacturing maintains files containing or refer to the location of objective evidence establishing the safety and effectiveness of the device as required by Annex 1 of the MDD. Verify that the manufacturer followed a defined and effective process to establish and maintain a file containing documents defining product specifications and quality system requirements for each newa and existing type/modes of medical devices. Since the last audit, has the manufacturer introduced new products in the EU? Has the manufacturer followed a defined and effective process to obtain an approval from the Notified Body to CE mark a product prior to selling it in the EU? (does not apply to class I devices)

7.2.2 Review of requirements related to the product	
	Does the organization review the requirements related to the product?
	Is this review conducted prior to the organization's commitment to supply a product to the customer (e.g. submission of tenders, acceptance of contracts or orders, acceptance of changes to contracts or orders)?
	Does the organization ensure that:
	a) Product requirements are defined and documented?
	b) Contract or order requirements differing from those previously expressed are resolved?
	c) The organization has the ability to meet the defined requirements?
	Are records of the results of the review and actions arising from the review maintained (see 4.2.4)?

Doc. Reference	Adequate?	Stage I (clauses marked *)	Stage II

	REQUIREMENTS	
	Where the customer provides no documented statement of requirement, are the customer requirements confirmed by the organization before acceptance?	
	Where product requirements are changed, does the organization ensure that relevant documents are amended and that relevant personnel are made aware of the changed requirements?	
7.2.3 Customer communication		
	Has the organization determined and implemented effective arrangements for communicating with customers in relation to:	
	a) Product information?	
	b) Enquiries, contracts or order handling, including amendments?	
	c) Customer feedback, including customer complaints? (see 8.2.1)	
	d) Advisory notices? (see 8.5.1)	
7.3 Design and development		
7.3.1 Design and/or development planning		
	Has the organization established documented procedures for design and development?	
	Does the organization plan and control the design and development of product?	
	During the design and development planning, does the organization determine:	
	a) The design and development stages?	
	b) The review, verification, validation and design transfer activities (see Note) that are appropriate at each design and development stage?	
	c) The responsibilities and authorities for design and development?	

Doc. Reference	Adequate?	Stage I (clauses marked *)	Stage II

	REQUIREMENTS
	Does the organization manage the interfaces between different groups involved in design and development to ensure effective communication and clear assignment of responsibility?
	Is planning output documented, and updated as appropriate, as the design and development progresses? (See 4.2.3)
Australia	Verify that effective planning for design and development is documented, typically as part of a Quality Plan [TG(MD)R Sch3 P1 Cl 4)1.4)].
7.3.2 Design and development inputs	
	Have inputs relating to product requirements been determined and records maintained (see 4.2.4)?
	Do these inputs include:
	a) Functional, performance and safety requirements, according to the intended use?
	b) Applicable statutory and regulatory requirements?
	c) Where applicable, information derived from previous similar designs?
	d) Other requirements essential for design and development?
	e) Output(s) of risk management (see 7.1)?
	Are these inputs reviewed for adequacy and approved?
	Are requirements complete, unambiguous and not in conflict with each other?
Australia	Verify that the manufacturer has identified the relevant Essential Principles that apply to the medical device [TG(MD)R Sch1 Essential Principles].
7.3.3 Design and development outputs	
	Are the outputs of design and development provided in a form that enables verification against the design and development input, and is it approved prior to release?

Doc. Reference	Adequate?	Stage I (clauses marked *)	Stage II

	REQUIREMENTS
	Do design and development outputs:
	a) meet the input requirements for design and development?
	b) Provide appropriate information for purchasing, production and for service provision?
	c) Contain or reference product acceptance criteria?
	d) Specify the characteristics of the product that are essential for its safe and proper use?
	Are records of the design and development outputs maintained (see 4.2.4)?
7.3.4 Design and development review	
	At suitable stages, are systematic reviews of design and development performed in accordance with planned arrangements (see 7.3.1):
	a) To evaluate the ability of the results of design and development to meet requirements?
	b) To identify any problems and propose necessary actions?
	Do participants in such reviews include representatives of functions concerned with the design and development stage(s) being reviewed, as well as other specialist personnel (see 5.5.1 and 6.2.1)?
	Are records of the results of the reviews and any necessary actions maintained (see 4.2.4)?
EU	Does the supplier evaluate the need for risk analysis throughout the design process and maintain records of any risk analysis performed? (MDD Annex 1)
7.3.5 Design and development verification	
	Is verification performed in accordance with planned arrangements (see 7.3.1) to ensure that the design and development outputs have met the design and development input requirements?
	Are records of the results of the verification and any necessary actions maintained?

Doc. Reference	Adequate?	Stage I (clauses marked *)	Stage II

	REQUIREMENTS
Australia	Confirm that documentation identifies whether relevant state of the art standards have been applied in full or in part. If standards have not been applied, ensure that the manufacturer has documented a rationale to explain why alternative methods have been applied to demonstrate compliance with the Essential Principles [TG(MD)R Sch3 Part 5)1.4)(c)(iii)(C)]. For devices incorporating a medicinal substance, verify that documentation also identifies the data to be derived from tests conducted in relation to the substance, and its interaction with the device [TG(MD)R Sch 3 Part 5)1.4)(c)(v)].
7.3.6 Design and development validation	
	Is design and development validation performed in accordance with planned arrangements (see 7.3.1) to ensure that the resulting product is capable of meeting the requirements for the specified application or intended use?
	Is validation completed prior to the delivery or implementation of the product (see Note 1)?
	Are records of the results of validation and any necessary actions maintained (see 4.2.4)?
	As part of design and development validation, does the organization perform clinical evaluations and/or evaluation of performance of the medical device, as required by national or regional regulations (see Note 2)?
Australia	Verify that records of the validation include clinical evidence as required by the clinical evidence procedures [TG(MD) Sch3 P1 Cl 5)1.4)(c)(vii) and TG(MD) Sch3 P8].
7.3.7 Control of design and development changes	
	Are design and development changes identified and records maintained?

Doc. Reference	Adequate?	Stage I (clauses marked *)	Stage II

	REQUIREMENTS
	Are changes reviewed, verified, and validated, as appropriate, and approved before implementation?
	Does the review of design and development changes include evaluation of the effect of the changes on constituent parts and product already delivered?
	Are records of the results of the review of changes and any necessary actions maintained?
Australia	Verify that the manufacturer has a process or procedure for notifying the auditing organization of a substantial change to the design process or the range of products to be manufactured [TG(MD)R Sch3 Cl1.5]. Verify that the manufacturer has a process or procedure for identifying a proposed substantial change to the design, or the intended performance, of a Class AIMD or Class III device, and to notify the assessment body prior to implementing the change [TG(MD)R Sch3 P1 Cl 4)1.6)].
EU	Do documented procedures identify the need to report essential changes to the Notified Body, (MDD Annex II, V, VI, 3.4)
7.4 Purchasing	
7.4.1 Purchasing process	
	Has the organization established documented procedures to ensure that purchased product conforms to specified purchase requirements?
	Is the type and extent of control applied to the supplier and the purchased product dependent upon the effect of the purchased product on subsequent product realization or the final product?
	Does the organization evaluate and select suppliers based on their ability to supply product in accordance with the organization's requirements?
	Have criteria for selection, evaluation and re-evaluation been established?

Doc. Reference	Adequate?	Stage I (clauses marked *)	Stage II

	REQUIREMENTS
	Are records of the results of evaluation and any necessary actions arising from the evaluation maintained (see 4.2.4)?
Australia	If the manufacturer outsources to the Australian Sponsor a quality management system requirement or an obligation on the manufacturer from the Australian regulations, verify that the manufacturer treats the Sponsor as a supplier and has adequate supplier controls for those activities. For example, making applications on behalf of the manufacturer to the TGA [TG Act s41EB], representing the manufacturer in interactions with the TGA [41FN(3)], adverse event reporting, as the first point for handling customer complaints, as an intermediary in recalls of products [TG(MD) Regs Schedule 3 - Part 3)1:1.4)], or in the notification of substantial changes to the quality management system or product range or the provision of records [TG(MD) Regs Schedule 3 - Part 1.9 ,1:1.5].
7.4.2 Purchasing information	
	Does purchasing information describe the product to be purchased, including where appropriate:
	a) Requirements for approval of product, procedures, processes and equipment?
	b) Requirements for qualification of personnel?
	c) Quality management system requirements?
	Does the organization ensure the adequacy of specified purchase requirements prior to their communication to the supplier?
	To the extent required for traceability given in 7.5.3.2, does the organization maintain relevant purchasing information, i.e. documents (see 4.2.3) and records (see 4.2.4)?
7.4.3 Verification of purchased product	
	Has the organization established and implemented the inspection or other activities necessary for ensuring that purchased product meets specified purchase requirements?

Doc. Reference	Adequate?	Stage I (clauses marked *)	Stage II

	REQUIREMENTS	
	Where the organization or its customer intends to perform verification at the supplier's premises, does the organization state the intended verification arrangements and method of product release in the purchasing information?	
	Are records of the verification maintained (see 4.2.4)?	
7.5 Production and service provision		
7.5.1 Control of production and service provision		
7.5.1.1 General Requirements		
	Does the organization plan and carry out production and service provision under controlled conditions?	
	Do the controlled conditions include, as applicable:	
	a) The availability of information that describes the characteristics of the product?	
	b) The availability of documented procedures, documented requirements, work instructions, reference materials and reference measurement procedures as necessary?	
	c) The use of suitable equipment?	
	d) The availability and use of monitoring and measuring devices?	
	e) The implementation of monitoring and measurement?	
	f) The implementation of release, delivery and post-delivery activities?	
	g) The implementation of defined operations for labeling and packaging?	
	Does the organization establish and maintain a record (see 4.2.4) for each batch of medical devices that provides traceability to the extent specified in 7.5.3 and identifies the amount manufactured and amount approved for distribution?	
	Is the batch record verified and approved?	
7.5.1.2 Control of production and service provision — Specific requirements		

Doc. Reference	Adequate?	Stage I (clauses marked *)	Stage II

	REQUIREMENTS

7.5.1.2.1 Cleanliness of product and contamination control	
	Does the organization establish documented requirements for cleanliness of product if:
	a) Product is cleaned by the organization prior to sterilization and/or its use, or
	b) Product is supplied non-sterile to be subjected to a cleaning process prior to sterilization and/or its use, or
	c) Product is supplied to be used non-sterile and its cleanliness is of significance in use, or
	d) Process agents are to be removed from product during manufacture?
	If product is cleaned in accordance with a) or b) above, the requirements contained in 6.4 a) and 6.4 b) do not apply prior to the cleaning process.
7.5.1.2.2 Installation activities	
	If appropriate, does the organization establish documented requirements which contain acceptance criteria for installing and verifying the installation of the medical device?
	If the agreed customer requirements allow installation to be performed other than by the organization or its authorized agent, does the organization provide documented requirements for installation and verification?
	Are records of installation and verification performed by the organization or its authorized agent maintained (see 4.2.4)?
7.5.1.2.3 Servicing activities	
	If servicing is a specified requirement, does the organization establish documented procedures, work instructions and reference materials and reference measurement procedures, as necessary, for performing servicing activities and verifying that they meet the specified requirements?

Doc. Reference	Adequate?	Stage I (clauses marked *)	Stage II

	REQUIREMENTS
	Are records of servicing activities carried out by the organization maintained (see 4.2.4)?
7.5.1.3 Particular requirements for sterile medical devices	
	Does the organization maintain records of the process parameters for the sterilization process which was used for each sterilization batch (see 4.2.4)?
	Are sterilization records traceable to each production batch of medical devices (see 7.5.1.1)?
7.5.2 Validation of processes for production and service provision	
7.5.2.1 General requirements	
	Does the organization validate any processes for production and service provision where the resulting output cannot be verified by subsequent monitoring or measurement? (this includes any processes where deficiencies become apparent only after the product is in use or the service has been delivered)
	Does validation demonstrate the ability of the processes to achieve planned results?
	Has the organization established arrangements for these processes including, as applicable:
	a) Defined criteria for review and approval of the processes?
	b) Approval of equipment and qualification of personnel?
	c) Use of specific methods and procedures?
	d) Requirements for records (see 4.2.4)?
	e) Re-validation?
	Has the organization established documented procedures for the validation of the application of computer software (and changes to such software and/or its application) for production and service provision that affect the ability of the product to conform to specified requirements?
	Are such software applications validated prior to initial use?
	Are records of validation maintained (see 4.2.4)?

Doc. Reference	Adequate?	Stage I (clauses marked *)	Stage II

	REQUIREMENTS
Australia	Confirm that methods of validation have regard to the generally acknowledged state of the art (e.g. current Medical Device Standard Orders - MDSO, ISO/IEC Standards, BP, EP, USP etc.) [TG Act s41CB, TG(MD)R Sch 1 P1)2 1)].
7.5.2.2 Particular requirements for sterile medical devices	
	Has the organization established documented procedures for the validation of sterilization processes?
	Are sterilization processes validated prior to initial use?
	Are records of validation of each sterilization process maintained (see 4.2.4)?
Australia	Verify that methods of sterilization validation have regard to the generally acknowledged state of the art (e.g. current Australian Medical Device Standard Orders - MDSO, ISO 11135, ISO 11137) [TG(MD)R Sch1 P1)2 1)].
7.5.3 Identification and traceability	
7.5.3.1 Identification	
	Does the organization identify the product by suitable means throughout product realization and does the organization establish documented procedures for such product identification?
	Has the organization established documented procedures to ensure that medical devices returned to the organization are identified and distinguished from conforming product [see 6.4 d)]?
7.5.3.2 Traceability	
7.5.3.2.1 General	
	Has the organization established documented procedures for traceability?
	Do such procedures define the extent of product traceability and the records required (see 8.3 ,4.2.4 and 8.5)?

Doc. Reference	Adequate?	Stage I (clauses marked *)	Stage II

	REQUIREMENTS
	Does the organization control and record the unique identification of the product, where traceability is a requirement (see 4.2.4)?
EU	Does the manufacturer have procedures identifying the requirements of labeling and instructions for use as defined in MDD, Annex 1 point 13, and is regulations for CE marking included in these procedures. (MDD 3, Article 17 and Annex 12).
	Are language requirements defined in procedures for the information identified in MDD, Annex 1point 13 for the applicable markets.
7.5.3.2.2 Particular requirements for active implantable medical devices and implantable medical devices	
	In defining the records required for traceability, does the organization include records of all components, materials and work environment conditions, if these could cause the medical device not to satisfy its specified requirements?
	Does the organization require that its agents or distributors maintain records of the distribution of medical devices to allow traceability and that such records be available for inspection?
	Are records of the name and address of the shipping package consignee maintained (see 4.2.4)?
7.5.3.3 Status identification	
	Does the organization identify the product status with respect to monitoring and measurement requirements?
	Is the identification of product status maintained throughout production, storage, installation and servicing of the product to ensure that only product that has passed the required inspections and tests (or released under an authorized concession) is dispatched, used or installed?
7.5.4 Customer property	

Doc. Reference	Adequate?	Stage I (clauses marked *)	Stage II

	REQUIREMENTS
	Does the organization exercise care with customer property while it is under the organization's control or being used by the organization?
	Does the organization identify, verify, protect and safeguard customer property provided for use or incorporation into the product?
	If any customer property is lost, damaged, or otherwise found to be unsuitable for use, is this reported to the customer and are records maintained (see 4.2.4)?
7.5.5 Preservation of product	
	Has the organization established documented procedures or documented work instructions for preserving the conformity of product during internal processing and delivery to the intended destination?
	Does this preservation include identification, handling, packaging, storage and protection, and also apply to the constituent parts of a product?
	Has the organization established documented procedures or documented work instructions for the control of product with a limited shelf-life or requiring special storage conditions?
	Are such special storage conditions controlled and recorded (see 4.2.4)?
7.6 Control of monitoring and measuring devices	
	Does the organization determine monitoring and measuring to be undertaken and the monitoring and measuring devices needed to provide evidence of conformity of product to determined requirements (guide reference 7.2.1)?
	Has the organization established documented procedures to ensure that monitoring and measurement can be carried out and are carried out in a manner that is consistent with the monitoring and measurement requirements?

Doc. Reference	Adequate?	Stage I (clauses marked *)	Stage II

	REQUIREMENTS
	Where necessary to ensure valid results, is measuring equipment:
	a) Calibrated or verified at specified intervals, or prior to use, against measurement standards traceable to international or national measurement standards; where no such standards exist, is the basis used for calibration or verification recorded?
	b) Adjusted or re-adjusted as necessary?
	c) Identified to enable the calibration status to be determined?
	d) Safeguarded from adjustments that would invalidate the measurement result?
	e) Protected from damage and deterioration during handling, maintenance and storage?
	Does the organization assess and record the validity of the previous measuring results when the equipment is found not to conform to requirements?
	Does the organization take appropriate action on the equipment and any product affected?
	Are records of the results of calibration and verification maintained (see 4.2.4)?
	When used in the monitoring and measurement of specified requirements, is the ability of computer software to satisfy the intended application confirmed prior to initial use and reconfirmed as necessary ?
8 Measurement, analysis and improvement	
8.1 General	

Doc. Reference	Adequate?	Stage I (clauses marked *)	Stage II

	REQUIREMENTS
	Does the organization plan and implement the monitoring, measurement, analysis and improvement processes needed:
	a) To demonstrate conformity of the product?
	b) To ensure conformity of the quality management system?
	c) To maintain the effectiveness of the quality management system?
	Does this include determination of applicable methods, including statistical techniques, and the extent of their use?
8.2 Monitoring and measurement	
8.2.1 Feedback	
	As one of the measurements of the performance of the quality management system, does the organization monitor information relating to whether the organization has met customer requirements?
	Have the methods for obtaining and using this information been determined?
	Has the organization established a documented procedure for a feedback system [see 7.2.3 c)] to provide early warning of quality problems and for input into the corrective and preventive action processes (see 8.5.2 and 8.5.3)?
	If national or regional regulations require the organization to gain experience from the post-production phase, does the review of this experience form part of the feedback system (see 8.5.1)?

Doc. Reference	Adequate?	Stage I (clauses marked *)	Stage II

	REQUIREMENTS
Australia	Verify that the organization has procedures for a post-marketing system that includes a systematic review of post-production experience (e.g. from; expert user groups, customer surveys, customer complaints and warranty claims, service and repair information, literature reviews, post-production clinical trials, user feedback other than complaints, device tracking and registration schemes, user reactions during training, adverse event reports). Investigation should take place in a timely manner to ensure that reporting timeframes for adverse events or advisory notices may be met [TG(MD)R Sch3 P3)1.4 1)(a)].
8.2.2 Internal audit	
	Does the organization conduct internal audits at planned intervals to determine whether the quality management system
	a) Conforms to the planned arrangements (see 7.1), to the requirements of this International Standard and to the quality management system requirements established by the organization?
	b) Is effectively implemented and maintained?
	Is an audit programme planned, taking into consideration the status and importance of the processes and areas to be audited, as well as the results of previous audits?
	Are the audit criteria, scope, frequency and methods defined?
	Does selection of auditors and conduct of audits ensure objectivity and impartiality of the audit process (e.g. auditors shall not audit their own work)?
	Are the responsibilities and requirements for planning and conducting audits, and for reporting results and maintaining records (see 4.2.4) defined in a documented procedure?

Doc. Reference	Adequate?	Stage I (clauses marked *)	Stage II

	REQUIREMENTS
	Does management responsible for the area being audited ensure that actions are taken without undue delay to eliminate detected nonconformities and their causes?
	Do follow-up activities include the verification of the actions taken and the reporting of verification results? (see 8.5.2)
8.2.3 Measurement and monitoring of processes	
	Does the organization apply suitable methods for monitoring and, where applicable, measurement of the quality management system processes?
	Do these methods demonstrate the ability of the processes to achieve planned results?
	When planned results are not achieved, is correction and corrective action taken, as appropriate, to ensure conformity of the product?
8.2.4 Monitoring and measurement of product	
8.2.4.1 General requirements	
	Does the organization monitor and measure the characteristics of the product to verify that product requirements have been met?
	Is this carried out at appropriate stages of the product realization process in accordance with the planned arrangements (see 7.1) and documented procedures (see 7.5.1.1)?
	Is evidence of conformity with the acceptance criteria maintained?
	Do records indicate the person(s) authorizing release of the product (see 4.2.4)?
	Does the organization ensure that product release and service delivery do not proceed until the planned arrangements (see 7.1) have been satisfactorily completed?
8.2.4.2 Particular requirement for active implantable medical devices and implantable medical devices	

Doc. Reference	Adequate?	Stage I (clauses marked *)	Stage II

	REQUIREMENTS
	Does the organization record (see 4.2.4) the identity of personnel performing any inspection or testing?
8.3 Control of nonconforming product	
	Does the organization ensure that product which does not conform to product requirements is identified and controlled to prevent its unintended use or delivery?
	Are the controls and related responsibilities and authorities for dealing with nonconforming product defined in a documented procedure?
	Does the organization deal with nonconforming product by one or more of the following ways?
	a) By taking action to eliminate the detected nonconformity
	b) By authorizing its use, release or acceptance under concession
	c) By taking action to preclude its original intended use or application
	Does the organization ensure that nonconforming product is accepted by concession only if regulatory requirements are met?
	Are records of the identity of the person(s) authorizing the concession maintained (see 4.2.4)?
	Are records of the nature of nonconformities and any subsequent actions taken, including concessions obtained maintained (see 4.2.4)?
	When nonconforming product is corrected, is it subject to re-verification to demonstrate conformity to the requirements?
	When nonconforming product is detected after delivery or use has started, does the organization take action appropriate to the effects, or potential effects, of the nonconformity?

Doc. Reference	Adequate?	Stage I (clauses marked *)	Stage II

	REQUIREMENTS
	If product needs to be reworked (one or more times), does the organization document the rework process in a work instruction that has undergone the same authorization and approval procedure as the original work instruction?
	Prior to authorization and approval of the work instruction, is a determination of any adverse effect of the rework upon product made and documented (see 4.2.3 and 7.5.1)?
8.4 Analysis of data	
	Does the organization establish documented procedures to determine, collect and analyse appropriate data to demonstrate the suitability and effectiveness of the quality management system and to evaluate if improvement of the effectiveness of the quality management system can be made?
	Does this include data generated as a result of monitoring and measurement and from other relevant sources?
	Does the analysis of data provide information relating to:
	a) Feedback (see 8.2.1)?
	b) Conformity to product requirements? (See 7.2.1)
	c) Characteristics and trends of processes and products including opportunities for preventive action?
	d) Suppliers?
	Are records of the results of the analysis of data maintained (see 4.2.4)?
8.5 Improvement	
8.5.1 General	
	Does the organization identify and implement any changes necessary to ensure and maintain the continued suitability and effectiveness of the quality management system through the use of the quality policy, quality objectives, audit results, analysis of data, corrective and preventive actions and management review?

Doc. Reference	Adequate?	Stage I (clauses marked *)	Stage II

	REQUIREMENTS
	Does the organization establish documented procedures for the issue and implementation of advisory notices and are these procedures capable of being implemented at any time?
Australia	Verify the manufacturer has implemented a post-marketing system that includes provisions for the recovery of devices. [Therapeutic Goods Act 41 ,1989FN(4) & (3) Therapeutic Goods (Medical Devices) Regulations – 2002 5.8 ,5.7, Sch3 Cl3)1.4)(c)(ii) TGA Uniform recall procedure for therapeutic goods (URPTG)]
EU	Are the procedures for Vigilance reporting in conformance with MDD Annex II, V, and VI (MEDDEV 1-2.12)
	Are records of all customer complaint investigations maintained (see 4.2.4)?
	If investigation determines that the activities outside the organization contributed to the customer complaint, is relevant information exchanged between the organizations involved (see 4.1)?
	If any customer complaint is not followed by corrective and/ or preventive action, is the reason authorized (see 5.5.1) and recorded (see 4.2.4)?
	If national or regional regulations require notification of adverse events that meet specific reporting criteria, does the organization establish documented procedures to such notification to regulatory authorities?
Australia	Verify that the Manufacturer has implemented a post-marketing system that includes provisions for adverse event reporting. [Therapeutic Goods Act 41 ,1989FN(4) & (3) Therapeutic Goods (Medical Devices) Regulations – 2002 5.8 ,5.7, Sch3 Cl3)1.4)(c)(i)]

Doc. Reference	Adequate?	Stage I (clauses marked *)	Stage II

	REQUIREMENTS
EU	Are procedures for the reporting of recall to the relevant competent authority and the NB compliant? (MDD, Annex II, V, VI, 3.1)
8.5.2 Corrective action	
	Does the organization take action to eliminate the cause of nonconformities in order to prevent recurrence and are corrective actions appropriate to the effects of the nonconformities encountered?
	Has a documented procedure been established to define requirements for:
	a) Reviewing nonconformities (including customer complaints)?
	b) Determining the causes of nonconformities?
	c) Evaluating the need for action to ensure that nonconformities do no recur?
	d) Determining and implementing action needed, including, if appropriate, updating documentation (see 4.2)?
	e) Recording of the results of any investigation and of action taken (see 4.2.4)?
	f) Reviewing the corrective action taken and its effectiveness?
8.5.3 Preventive action	
	Does the organization determine action to eliminate the causes of potential nonconformities in order to prevent their occurrence and are preventive actions appropriate to the effects of the potential problems?

Doc. Reference	Adequate?	Stage I (clauses marked *)	Stage II

	REQUIREMENTS
	Has a documented procedure been established to define requirements for:
	a) Determining potential nonconformities and their causes?
	b) Evaluating the need for action to prevent occurrence of nonconformities?
	c) Determining and implementing action needed?
	d) Recording of the results of any investigations and of action taken (see 4.2.4)?
	e) Reviewing preventive action taken and its effectiveness?

Doc. Reference	Adequate?	Stage I (clauses marked *)	Stage II

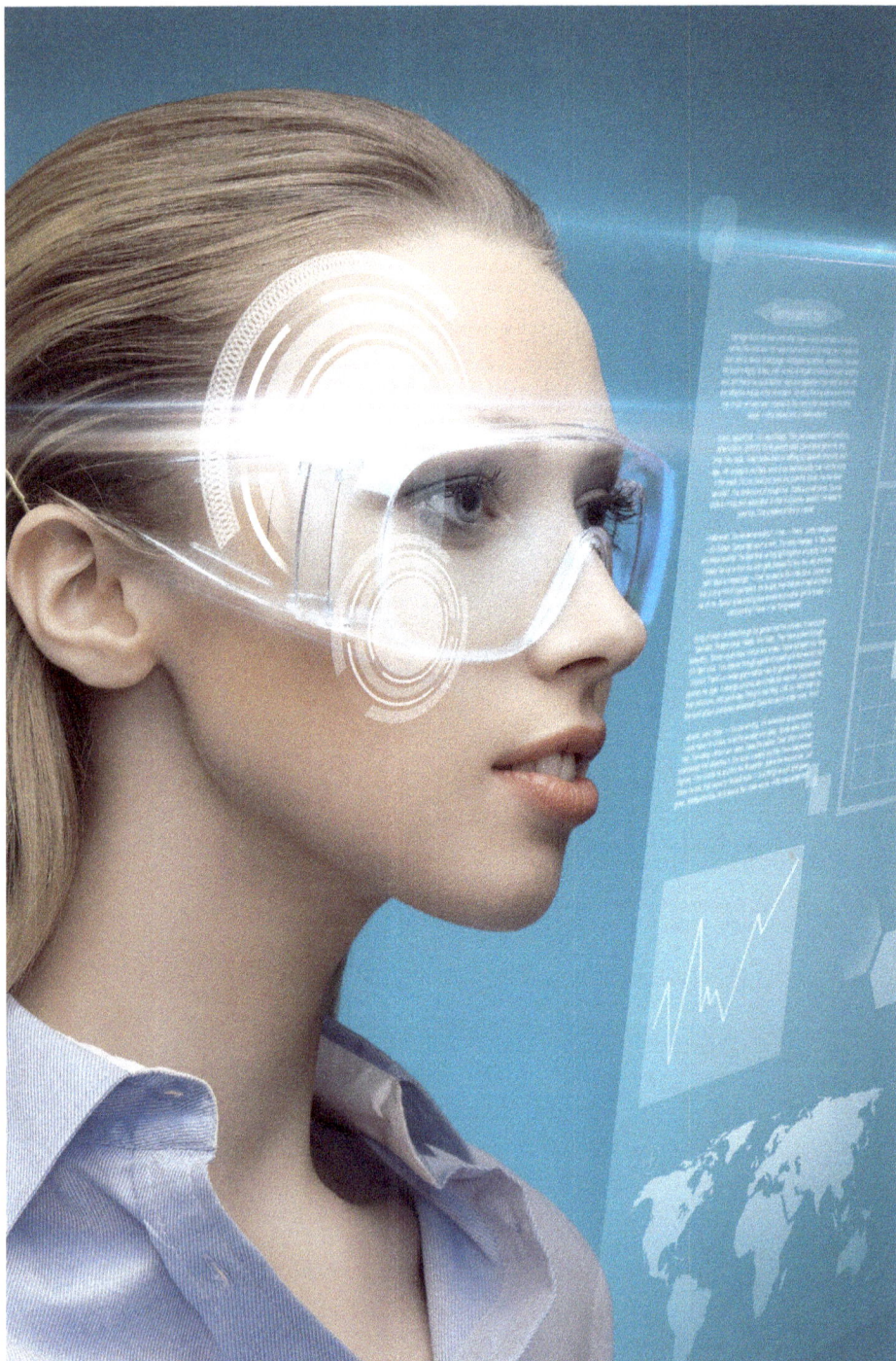

MDSAP
ISO 13485 Requirements &

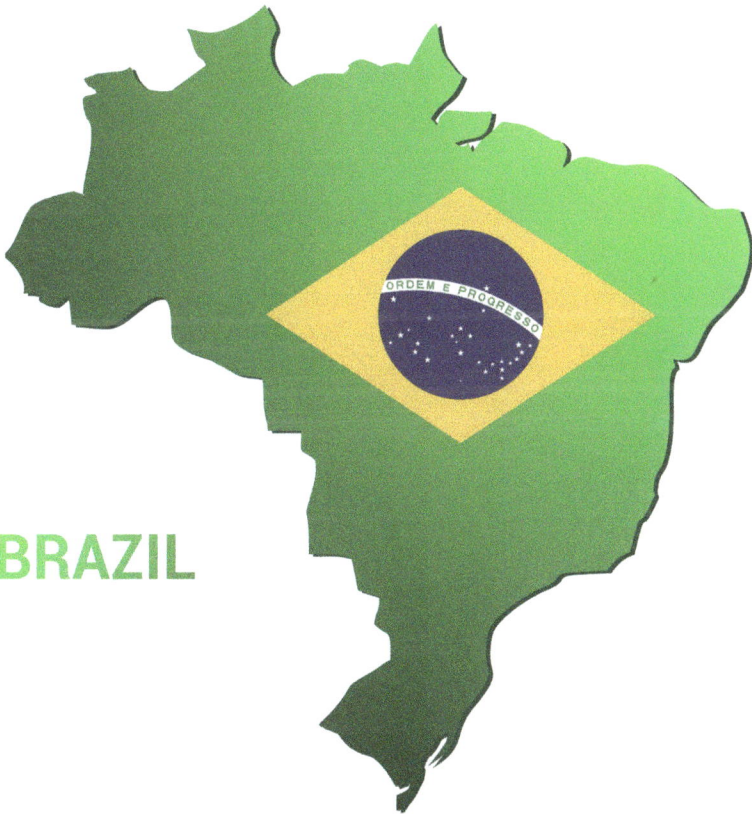

BRAZIL

Management

The intent of the Management Process is to provide adequate resources for device design, manufacturing, quality assurance, distribution, installation, and servicing activities; to assure the quality management system is functioning properly and effectively; and to monitor the quality management system and make necessary adjustments. A quality management system that has been implemented effectively and is monitored to identify and address existing and potential problems is more likely to produce medical devices that function as intended.

The management representative is responsible for ensuring that the requirements of the quality management system have been effectively defined, documented, implemented, and maintained. Prior to the audit of a process, it may be helpful to interview the management representative (or designee) to obtain an overview of the process and a feel for management's knowledge and understanding of the process.

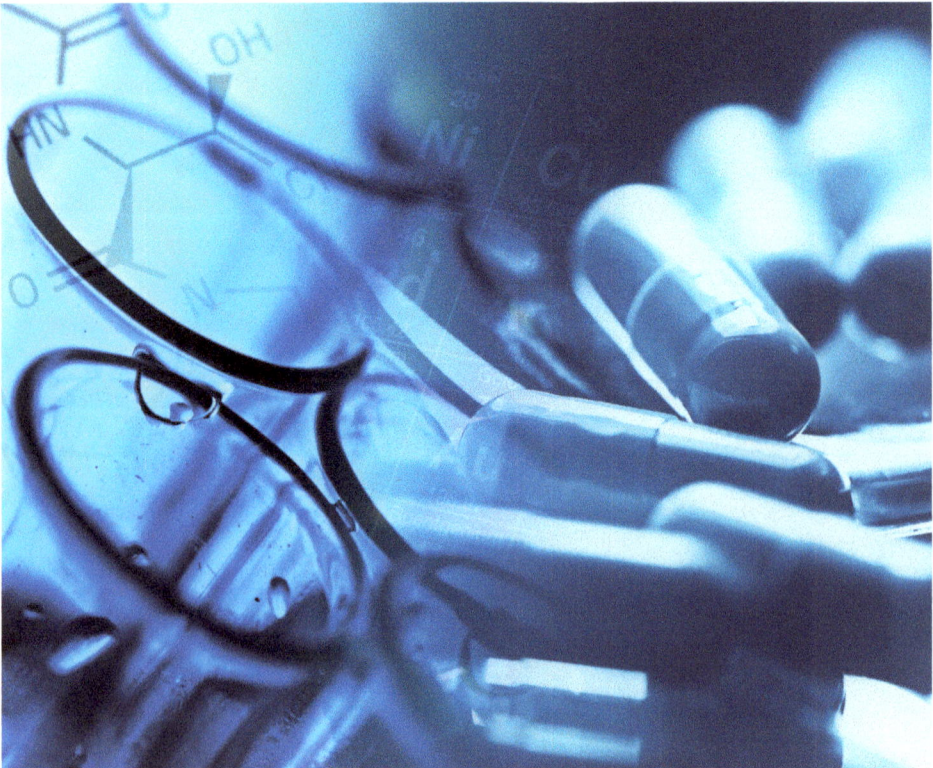

Clause and Regulation:
ISO 13485:2016: 4.1.1, 4.1.2, 4.1.3, 4.2.2, 4.1.4, 5.4.2;
ANVISA: RDC ANVISA 16/2013: 2.1, 5.6;
ANVISA: RDC ANVISA 16/2013: 2.2.5

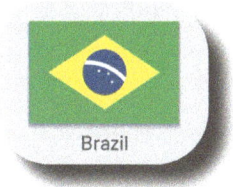

Brazil

Confirm that the manufacturer ensures that any consultant who gives advice regarding design, purchasing, manufacturing, packaging, labeling, storage, installation, or servicing of medical devices has proper qualification to perform such tasks. Those consultants shall be contracted as a formal service supplier, according to purchasing controls defined by the manufacturer [RDC ANVISA 16/2013: 2.3.3].

A review of employee training records can be performed to ensure that employees have been trained regarding the medical device organization's quality policy and objectives. In particular, this should be done for employees involved in key operations that affect product realization and product quality.

During the audit of the Production and Service Controls process, ensure that employees who are involved in key operations that affect product realization and product quality have been trained in their specific job tasks, as well as the quality policy and objectives.
When appropriate, review the training records for those employees whose activities have contributed to process nonconformities.

When appropriate, assess the role of top management when risk-based decisions are made that appear to justify levels of risk that do not meet the medical device organization's previously established risk- acceptance criteria.

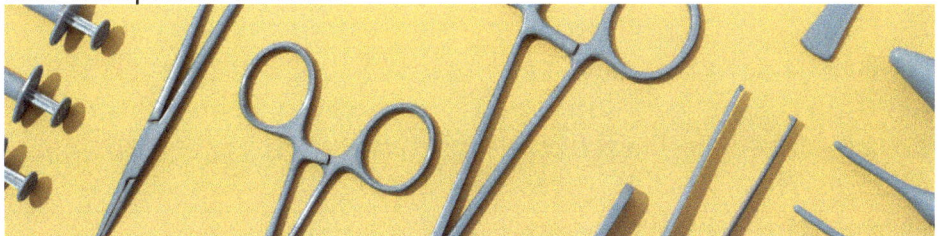

Device Marketing Authorization and Facility Registration
The Device Marketing Authorization and Facility Registration process may be audited as a linkage from the Management process and/or the Design and Development process.

Good Manufacturing Practices in Brazil

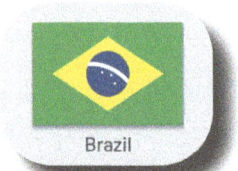

Manufacturer means any person who designs, manufactures, assembles or processes finished devices, including those who only perform sterilization process, labeling and packaging [RDC ANVISA 16/2013: 1.2.9].

For a domestic manufacturer, confirm that the establishment has ANVISA's authorization to manufacture medical devices (AFE - Autorização de Funcionamento da Empresa). For domestic and international manufacturers, verify that the products already distributed in the Brazilian market are registered/notified with ANVISA [Brazilian Federal Law nº 6360/76].

According Brazilian Legislation, the Good Manufacturing Practice (GMP) certification is a prerequisite for medical device registration. Therefore, the facility site inspection precedes the device registration request. Medical devices subject to notification do not need the GMP certificate, but even not being certified, their manufacturers shall comply with the GMP requirements.

Device marketing authorization shall be requested to ANVISA by the domestic manufacturer or importer (legal representative) formally established in Brazil. Registration is a comprehensive process for market authorization, applied to medical devices in classes III and IV. [ANVISA RDC nº 36/2015, RDC nº 40/2015]

Notification is a simplified market authorization process, applied to all medical device classes I and II. [ANVISA RDC nº 36/2015, RDC nº 40/2015]. Registration is valid for 10 years, while notification has no expiry date. Renewal of the registration shall be requested upon time defined at Brazilian Law 6360/1976.

Measurement, Analysis and Improvement

One of the most important activities in the quality management system is the identification of existing and potential causes of product and quality problems. Such causes must be identified so that appropriate and effective corrective or preventive actions can take place. These activities are carried out under the Measurement, Analysis and Improvement process.

Clause and Regulation
ISO: ISO 13485:2016: 4.2.1, 8.1, 8.2.1, 8.2.6, 8.5
ANVISA: RDC ANVISA 16/2013: 5.3.1, 7.1, 7.2

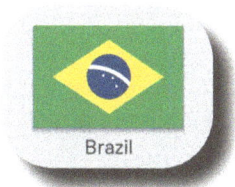

Brazil

Verify that the manufacturer has ensured that information about quality problems or nonconforming products are properly disseminated to those directly involved in the maintenance of product quality and to prevent occurrence of such problems [RDC ANVISA 16/2013: 7.1.1.6].

Verify that each manufacturer has established and maintains procedures to receive, examine, evaluate, investigate and document complaints. Such procedures must ensure that:

- Complaints are received, documented, analyzed, evaluated, investigated and documented by a formally designated unit
- Where applicable, complaints must be reported to the competent health authority
- Complaints must be examined to determine whether an investigation is necessary. When an investigation is not done, the unit must maintain a record that includes the reason that the investigation was not performed and the name of the persons responsible for the decision. Each manufacturer must examine, evaluate and investigate all complaints involving possible nonconformities of the product. Any claim for death, injury or threat to public health must be immediately reviewed, evaluated and investigated.
- The records of the investigation must include:

Product name, Date of receipt of the complaint, Any control number used, Name, address and telephone number of the complainant Nature of complaint, Data and research results [RDC ANVISA 16/2013: 7.2].

Medical Device Adverse Events and Advisory Notices Reporting
The Medical Device Adverse Events and Advisory Notices Reporting
process may be audited as a linkage from the Measurement, Analysis
and Improvement process.

Clause and Regulation
ISO: ISO 13485:2016: 4.2.1, 7.2.3, 8.2.2, 8.2.3
[RDC ANVISA 67/2009 – Art. 6°]

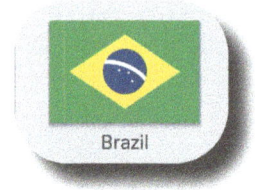

Brazil

Verify that a post-market surveillance system is established and
implemented in the medical device organization and integrated into
the Quality System, with procedures and work flows established to
ensure the correct and the prompt identification of adverse events,
the performance of investigations and use of the results to improve
the safety and effectiveness of the device when necessary
[RDC ANVISA 67/2009 – Art. 6°].
For domestic manufacturers (also applies to legal representatives in
Brazil) - verify that top management has designated a professional to be responsible for the post-market surveillance system. This
designation shall be documented
[RDC ANVISA 67/2009 – Art. 5°].
Verify that the medical device organization has mechanisms for
processing and recording complaints, conducting investigations,
and providing feedback directly to the complainant, or in the case
of an international manufacturer, to their legal representative in
Brazil, as necessary
[RDC ANVISA 67/2009 – Art. 6°, Art. 7°, Art. 9°].
Verify that the medical device organization has notified the regulatory authority about problems associated with their devices, including adverse events (critical or non-critical), any technical defect
that was identified regarding products already marketed, anything
that can cause a serious hazard to public health, or cases of counterfeit
[RDC ANVISA 67/2009 – Art. 8°].

For international manufacturer, verify that the legal representative in Brazil is aware about the occurrence of possibility of death, serious hazard to public health or cases of counterfeit, associated with their products exported to Brazil
[RDC ANVISA 67/2009 – Art. 8º].

Verify that procedures and work flows were established in order to identify when field actions (recalls and corrections) are necessary, in accordance with the medical device organization's post-market surveillance system and quality system [RDC ANVISA 67/2009 - Art. 6º, RDC ANVISA 23/2012 – Art. 1º, Art. 5º].

Verify that the medical device organization keeps records regarding field actions performed, including those that do not need to be reported to regulatory authorities [RDC ANVISA 23/2012 – Art. 4º; Art. 6º, Art. 10, Art. 11, Art. 16].

For domestic manufacturers (also applies to legal representatives in Brazil) - verify that the medical device organization has sent to the regulatory authority the reports requested, according Brazilian regulation [RDC ANVISA 23/2012– Art. 10, Art. 11].

Verify that the medical device organization has performed field actions based on potential or concrete evidence that their product does not comply with essential requirements of safety and effectiveness [RDC ANVISA 23/2012 – Art. 4º, Art. 6º, Art. 7º, Art. 13, Art. 14, Art. 15].

For domestic manufacturers (also applies to legal representatives in Brazil) - verify that the medical device organization has performed field actions when required by the regulatory authority [RDC ANVISA 23/2012 – Art. 6º].

For domestic manufacturers (also applies to legal representatives in Brazil) - verify that the medical device organization notified the regulatory authority regarding field actions, in accordance with requirements and deadlines established per Brazilian regulation
[RDC ANVISA 23/2012 – Art. 7º, Art. 8º].

For international manufacturers, verify that the legal representative in Brazil was aware about the occurrence of field actions performed on products exported to Brazil
[RDC ANVISA 67/2009 – Art. 8º].

RISK
MANAGEMENT

IDENTIFY THREATS

ASSESS VULNERABILITY

DETERMINE RISK

IDENTIFY MEASURES

PRIORITIZE RISK REDUCTION

Design and Development
The purpose of the Design and Development process is to control the design of a medical device and to assure that the device meets user needs, intended use, and its specified requirements. Attention to design and development planning, identifying design inputs, developing design outputs, verifying that design outputs meet design inputs, validating the design, controlling design changes, reviewing design results, transferring the design to production, and compiling the appropriate records will help a medical device organization assure that resulting designs will meet user needs, intended uses, and requirements. Review of the Design and Development process will also provide an opportunity to evaluate how the medical device organization has utilized risk management activities to ensure design inputs are comprehensive and meet user needs, to confirm that risk control measures that were planned have been implemented in the design, and to verify that risk control measures are effective in controlling or reducing risk.

Clause and Regulation
ISO: ISO 13485:2016: 4.1.1, 4.2.1, 7.1, 7.3.10
[RDC ANVISA 16/2013: 4.1.7, 4.2].

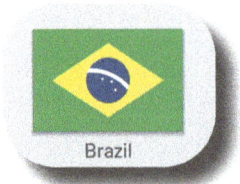

Brazil

According to Brazilian legislations, there is no exception to design control.
If design activities are outsourced, verify that the manufacturer has a complete device master record for the device and records of the design transfer to production
[RDC ANVISA 16/2013: 4.1.7, 4.2]. [RDC ANVISA 16/2013: 4.1.2, 4.1.11]
Verify that the manufacturer has established and maintains a continuous process of risk management which covers the entire life cycle of the product. Possible hazards must be identified in both normal and fault conditions, including those arising from human factors issues. The risk associated with those hazards, shall be calculated. Risks must be analyzed, evaluated and controlled, as necessary. Effectiveness of risk controls implemented shall be evaluated [RDC ANVISA 56/2001, RDC ANVISA 16/2013: 2.4].

Production and Service Controls

The purpose of the Production and Service Controls process is to manufacture products that meet specifications. Developing processes that are adequate to produce devices that meet specifications, validating (or fully verifying the results of) those processes, and monitoring and controlling those processes are all steps that help assure the result will be devices that meet specified requirements. After completing the audit of the medical device organization's Production and Service Controls process, the audit team will return to the Management process to make a final decision of whether top management ensures that an adequate and effective quality management system has been established and maintained at the medical device organization.

Clause and Regulation
ISO: ISO 13485:2016: 7.1, 7.2.1, 7.5.1
RDC ANVISA 16/2013: 2.2.1, 2.4, 4.1.2, 4.1.7, 5.1

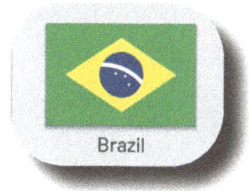

Brazil

Confirm that a pest control program has been established and where chemicals are used as part of the pest control program, the company must ensure that they do not affect product quality [RDC ANVISA 16/2013: 5.1.3.4].

Verify that the manufacturer has established and maintains housekeeping procedures and schedules for production areas and warehouses, in conformance with production specifications [RDC ANVISA 16/2013: 5.1.3.1].

Verify that analytical methods, supporting auxiliary systems for production and environmental control that can adversely affect product quality or the quality system are validated, periodically reviewed and, when necessary, revalidated according to documented procedures
[RDC ANVISA 16/2013: 5.5.2, 5.5.3].

Reviewing a validation
During review of a validation study, determine when applicable whether:

- The instruments used to generate the data were properly calibrated and maintained
- Predetermined product and process specifications were established
- Sampling plans used to collect test samples are based on a statistically valid rationale
- Data demonstrates predetermined specifications were met consistently
- Process tolerance limits were challenged
- Process equipment was properly installed, adjusted, and maintained
- Process monitoring instruments were properly calibrated and maintained
- Changes to the validated process were appropriately challenged (if applicable)
- Process operators were appropriately qualified.

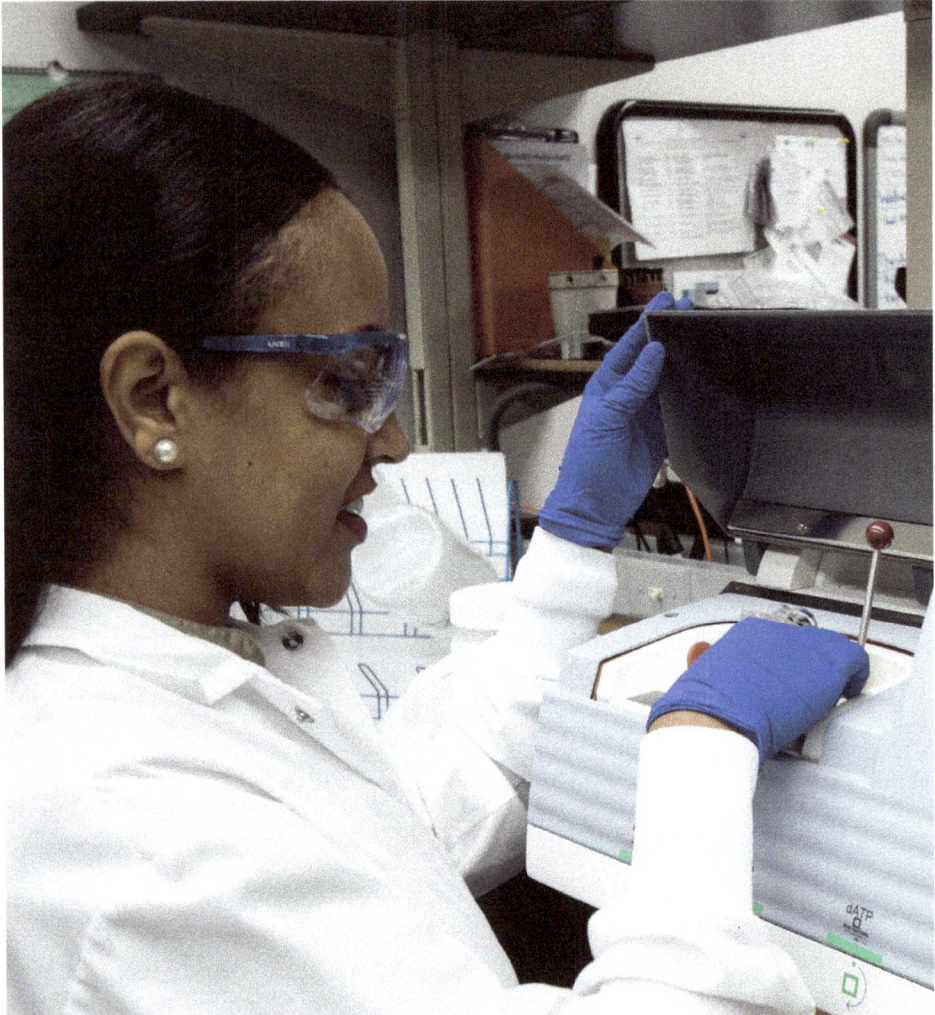

Purchasing

The intent of the Purchasing process is to ensure that purchased, sub-contracted, or otherwise received products and services conform to specified requirements. The medical device organization is expected to establish and maintain documented controls for planning and performing purchasing activities. The controls necessary depend on the effect of the product on the quality, safety, and effectiveness of the finished device. Effective purchasing processes incorporate purchasing requirements and specifications, the selection of acceptable suppliers based on the capability of the suppliers to provide acceptable product, the performance of necessary acceptance activities, and maintenance of the required quality records.

The management representative is responsible for ensuring that the requirements of the quality management system have been effectively defined, documented, implemented, and maintained. Prior to the audit of a process, it may be helpful to interview the management representative to obtain an overview of the process and a feel for management's knowledge and understanding of the process.

Clause and Regulation
ISO: ISO: ISO 13485:2016: 4.1.2, 4.1.3, 4.1.5, 7.1, 7.4.1, 7.4.2, 7.4.3
ANVISA: RDC ANVISA16/2013: 2.5.1, 2.4

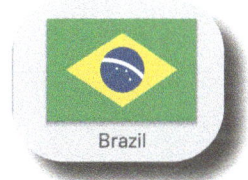

Brazil

Planning

In planning product realization, the medical device organization must determine as appropriate the quality objectives and requirements for the purchased products, the processes, documents, and resources specific to the purchased products, the criteria for purchased product acceptance, and the required verification, monitoring, inspection, and test activities specific to the purchased products. Planning of product realization often begins in the design and development of the product, including the translation of the design into production specifications. The translation of the design into production specifications includes the establishment of specified requirements for purchased product.

Quality objectives

Quality objectives are typically expressed as a measurable target or goal. The planning of product realization should include consideration of how the purchased product, the criteria for purchased product acceptance, and the required verification, monitoring, inspection, and test activities specific to the purchased product will achieve the quality objectives.

- Some examples of QOB include:
- Number of complaints -v- number of parts shipped
- On-time delivery %
- Supplier parts rejected
- Comparison of internal audit findings -v- external audit findings
- Achieving a certain accuracy if you're developing product - based software
- Annual Post-market surveillance
- Auditing our system for regulatory compliance

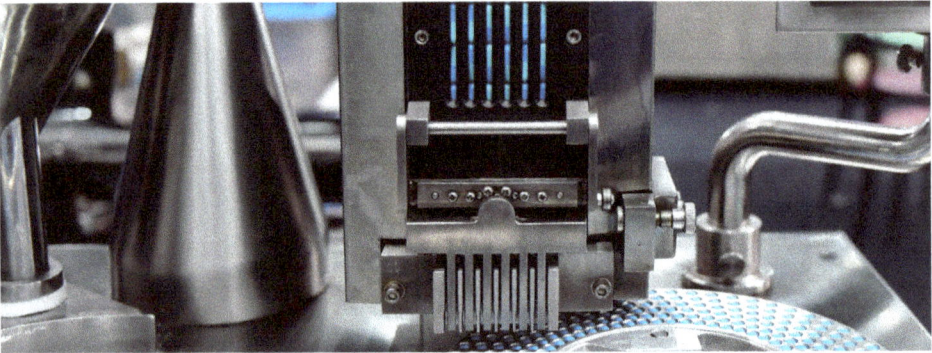

Some managers believe that the reward for hard work should be a paycheck. That's sort of like telling your children that they get to eat for doing something you're proud of. Employees are not children, but you are responsible for developing them into more valuable employees so that they can be promoted. If there is no incentive, your team will not be engaged. Therefore, pick a reward that is proportional to the bottom-line impact. Five percent of the bottom-line impact is what I like to target, but you would be amazed at how effective a few small rewards at each milestone can be. If you have trouble getting management approval for rewards, remind your boss of the bottom-line impact and link the rewards closely to the impact.

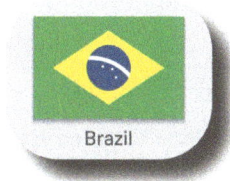

MDSAP
Audit Checklist

	REQUIREMENTS

4 Quality management system	

4.1 General requirements	
	Has the organization:
	a) identified the processes needed for the quality management system and their application throughout the organization (see 1.2)?
	b) determined the sequence and interaction of these processes?
	c) determined criteria and methods needed to ensure that both the operation and control of these processes are effective?
	d) ensured the availability of resources and information necessary to support the operation and monitoring of their processes?
	e) monitored, measured, and analyzed these processes
	f) implemented actions necessary to achieve planned results and maintain the effectiveness of these processes?
	Does the organization manage these processes in accordance with the requirements of this International Standard?
	Where an organization chooses to outsource any process that affects product conformity with requirements, does the organization ensure control over such processes?
	Is the control of such outsourced processes identified within the quality management system? (see 8.5.1)
4.2.1 General	

Doc. Reference	Adequate?	Stage I (clauses marked *)	Stage II
	Y/N	Initial›s	Initial›s

	REQUIREMENTS
	Does the quality management system documentation include:
	a) documented statements of a quality policy and quality objectives?
	b) a quality manual?
	c) documented procedures required by this international standard?
	d) documents needed by the organization to ensure the effective planning, operation and control of its processes?
	e) records required by this International Standard (see 4.2.4)?
	f) any other documentation specified by national or regional regulations?
	Has the organization established and maintained a file for each type or model of medical device either containing or identifying documents defining product specifications and quality system requirements (see 4.2.3)?
	Do these documents define the complete manufacturing process and, if applicable, installation and servicing?
Brazil	According to Brazilian legislations, there is no exception to design control. If design activities are outsourced, verify that the manufacturer has a complete device master record for the device and records of the design transfer to production [RDC ANVISA 4.2 ,4.1.7 :2013/16].
Brazil	Verify that the manufacturer maintains distribution records which include or make reference to: the name and address of the consignee, the identification and quantity of products shipped, the date of dispatch, and any numerical control used for traceability [RDC ANVISA 6.3 :2013/16].

Doc. Reference	Adequate?	Stage I (clauses marked *)	Stage II
		*	

	REQUIREMENTS
EU	Does the file contain or refer to the location of objective evidence establishing the safety and effectiveness of the device as required by Annex 1 of the MDD? (MDD Annex I)
4.2.2 Quality manual	
	Has the organization established and maintained a quality manual that includes:
	a) the scope of the quality management system, including details of and justification for any exclusion and/or non-application (see 1.2)?
	b) the documented procedures established for the quality management system, or reference to them?
	c) a description of the interaction between the processes of the quality management system?
	Does the quality manual outline the structure of the documentation used in the quality management system?
Brazil	For domestic manufacturers, confirm that the establishment has ANVISA's authorization to manufacture medical devices (AFE - Autorização de Funcionamento da Empresa.)
	For domestic and international manufacturers, verify that the products already distributed in the Brazilian market, are registered/notified with ANVISA [Brazilian Federal Law 76/6360].
EU	Are the applicable sections of the Medical Device Directive (MDD) included in the specified requirements throughout the documented quality system? Interpretation: A statement only indicating compliance/conformity with the relevant international or EU regulatory requirements is not acceptable.
4.2.3 Control of documents	
	Are documents required by the quality management system controlled?

Doc. Reference	Adequate?	Stage I (clauses marked *)	Stage II

	REQUIREMENTS
	Is a documented procedure established to define the controls needed:
	a) To review and approve documents for adequacy prior to issue?
	b) To review and update as necessary and re-approve documents?
	c) To ensure that changes and the current revision status of documents are identified?
	d) To ensure that relevant versions of applicable documents are available at points of use?
	e) To ensure the documents remain legible and readily identifiable?
	f) To ensure that documents of external origin are identified and their distribution controlled?
	g) To prevent the unintended use of obsolete documents and to apply suitable identification to them if they are retained for any purpose?
	Does the organization ensure that changes to documents are reviewed and approved either by the original approving function or another designated function which has access to pertinent background information upon which to base its decisions?
	Does the organization define the period for which at least one copy of obsolete controlled documents shall be retained?
	Does this period ensure that documents to which medical devices have been manufactured and tested are available for at least the lifetime of the medical device as defined by the organization, but not less than the retention period of any resulting record (see 4.2.4), or as specified by relevant regulatory requirements?

Doc. Reference	Adequate?	Stage I (clauses marked *)	Stage II

	REQUIREMENTS
Brazil	Verify that change records include a description of the change, identification of the affected documents, the signature of the approving individual(s), the approval date, and when the change becomes effective [RDC ANVISA 3.1.5 :2013/16]. Confirm that the manufacturer maintains a master list of the approved and effective documents [RDC ANVISA :2013/16 3.1.5]. Verify that electronic records and documents have backups [RDC ANVISA 3.1.6 :2013/16].
4.2.4 Control of quality records	
	Are records established and maintained to provide evidence of conformity to requirements and of the effective operation of the quality management system?
	Do records remain legible, readily identifiable and retrievable?
	Has a documented procedure been established to define the controls needed for the identification, storage, protection, retrieval, retention time and disposition of records?
	Does the organization retain the records for a period of time at least equivalent to the lifetime of the medical device as defined by the organization, but not less than two years from the date of product release by the organization or as specified by relevant regulatory requirements?
EU	Has the manufacturer retained for a period ending at least five years after the last product has been manufactured, the records listed in Annex II, 6.1 or Annex V, 5.1 or Annex VI, 5.1 (whichever applies)
5 Management responsibility	
5.1 Management commitment	

Doc. Reference	Adequate?	Stage I (clauses marked *)	Stage II

	REQUIREMENTS
	Has top management provided evidence of its commitment to the development and implementation of the quality management system and maintaining its effectiveness by:
	a) Communicating to the organization the importance of meeting customer as well as statutory and regulatory requirements?
	b) Establishing the quality policy?
	c) Ensuring that quality objectives are established?
	d) Conducting management reviews?
	e) Ensuring the availability of resources?
5.2 Customer focus	
	Does top management ensure that customer requirements are determined and met (see 7.2.1 and 8.2.1)?
5.3 Quality policy	
	Does top management ensure that the quality policy
	a) Is appropriate to the purpose of the organization?
	b) Includes a commitment to comply with requirements and to maintain the effectiveness of the quality management system?
	c) Provides a framework for establishing and reviewing quality objectives?
	d) Is communicated and understood within the organization?
	e) Is reviewed for continuing suitability?
5.4 Planning	
5.4.1 Quality objectives	
	Does top management ensure that quality objectives, including those needed to meet requirements for product (see 7.1a), are established at relevant functions and levels within the organization?
	Are quality objectives measurable?

Doc. Reference	Adequate?	Stage I (clauses marked *)	Stage II

	REQUIREMENTS
	Are quality objectives consistent with the quality policy?
5.4.2 Quality management system planning	
	Has top management ensured that:
	a) The planning of the quality management system is carried out in order to meet the requirements given in 4.1, as well as the quality objectives?
	b) The integrity of the quality management system is maintained when changes to the quality management system are planned and implemented?
5.5 Responsibility, authority and communication	
5.5.1 Responsibility and authority	
	Has top management ensured that responsibilities and authorities were defined, documented and communicated within the organization?
	Has top management established the interrelation of all personnel who manage, perform and verify work affecting quality, and ensured the independence and authority necessary to perform these tasks?
5.5.2 Management representative	
	Has top management appointed a member of management who, irrespective of other responsibilities, has responsibility and authority that includes:
	a) Ensuring that processes needed for the quality management system are established, implemented, and maintained?
	b) Reporting to top management on the performance of the quality management system and any need for improvement (see 8.5)?
	c) Ensuring the promotion of awareness of regulatory and customer requirements throughout the organization?
5.5.3 Internal communication	

Doc. Reference	Adequate?	Stage I (clauses marked *)	Stage II

	REQUIREMENTS
	Has top management ensured that appropriate communication processes have been established within the organization and that communication takes place regarding the effectiveness of the quality management system?
5.6 Management review	
5.6.1 General	
	Does top management review the organization's quality management system, at planned intervals, to ensure its continuing suitability, adequacy and effectiveness?
	Does this review include assessing opportunities for improvement and the need for changes to the quality management system, including the quality policy and quality objectives?
	Are records from management reviews maintained (see 4.2.4)?
5.6.2 Review input	
	Does the input to management review include information on:
	a) Results of audits?
	b) Customer feedback?
	c) Process performance and product conformity?
	d) Status of preventive and corrective actions?
	e) Follow-up actions from previous management reviews?
	f) Changes that could affect the quality management system?
	g) Recommendations for improvement?
	h) New or revised regulatory requirements?
Brazil	Confirm that relevant information about quality problems is identified and corrective and preventive actions are submitted to executive management for information and monitoring, as well as the competent health authority, if applicable [RDC ANVISA 7.1.1.7 :2013/16].

Doc. Reference	Adequate?	Stage I (clauses marked *)	Stage II

	REQUIREMENTS
5.6.3 Review output	
	Does output from the management review include any decisions and actions related to:
	a) Improvements needed to maintain the effectiveness of the quality management system and its processes?
	b) Improvement of product related to customer requirements?
	c) Resource needs?
6 Resource management	
6.1 Provision of resources	
	Does the organization determine and provide the resources needed:
	a) To implement the quality management system and to maintain its effectiveness?
	b) To meet regulatory and customer requirements?
6.2 Human resources	
6.2.1 General	
	Are personnel performing work affecting product quality competent on the basis of appropriate education, training, skills and experience?
6.2.2 Competence, awareness and training	

Doc. Reference	Adequate?	Stage I (clauses marked *)	Stage II

	REQUIREMENTS
	Does the organization:
	a) determine the necessary competence for personnel performing work affecting product quality?
	b) Provide training or take other actions to satisfy these needs?
	c) Evaluate the effectiveness of actions taken?
	d) Ensure that its personnel are aware of the relevance and importance of their activities and how they contribute to the achievement of the quality objectives?
	e) Maintain appropriate records of education, training, skills and experience (see 4.2.4)?
Brazil	Confirm that the manufacturer ensures that any consultant who gives advice regarding design, purchasing, manufacturing, packaging, labeling, storage, installation, or servicing of medical devices has proper qualification to perform such tasks. Those consultants shall be contracted as a formal service supplier, according to purchasing controls defined by the manufacturer [RDC ANVISA 2.3.3 :2013/16].
6.3 Infrastructure	
	Does the organization determine, provide and maintain the infrastructure needed to achieve conformity to product requirements?
	Infrastructure includes, as applicable:
	a) Buildings, workspace and associated utilities
	b) Process equipment, both hardware and software
	c) Supporting services such as transport or communication
	Does the organization establish documented requirements for maintenance activities, including their frequency, when such activities or lack thereof can affect product quality?
	Are records of such maintenance maintained (see 4.2.4)?

Doc. Reference	Adequate?	Stage I (clauses marked *)	Stage II

	REQUIREMENTS
Brazil	Verify that manufacturing facilities are configured in order to provide adequate means for production, avoid mix-ups or contamination of components, raw materials, in process products and finished devices; and to ensure the correct handling of the devices and production flow [RDC ANVISA 5.1.2 :2013/16].
	Has the organization determined and does it manage the work environment needed to achieve conformity to product requirements?
	a) Has the organization established documented requirements for health, cleanliness and clothing of personnel if contact between such personnel and the product or work environment could adversely affect the quality of the product (see 7.5.1.2.1)?
	b) If work environment conditions can have an adverse effect on product quality, has organization established documented requirements for the work environment conditions and documented procedures or work instructions to monitor and control these work environment conditions (see 7.5.1.2.1)?
	c) Does the organization ensure that all personnel who are required to work temporarily under special environmental conditions within the work environment are appropriately trained or supervised by a trained person [see 6.2.2 b)]?
	d) If appropriate, are special arrangements established and documented for the control of contaminated or potentially contaminated product in order to prevent contamination of other product, the work environment or personnel (see 7.5.3.1)?
Brazil	Verify that biosafety standards are used, when applicable [RDC ANVISA 5.1.3.6 :2013/16].

Doc. Reference	Adequate?	Stage I (clauses marked *)	Stage II
NA			

	REQUIREMENTS

7 Product realization	
7.1 Planning of product realization	
	Has the organization planned and developed the processes needed for product realization?
	Is the planning of product realization consistent with the requirements of the other processes of the quality management system (see 4.1)?
	In planning product realization, has the organization determined the following, as appropriate:
	a) Quality objectives and requirements for products?
	b) The need to establish processes, documents, and provide resources specific to the product?
	c) Required verification, validation, monitoring, inspection and test activities specific to the product and the criteria for product acceptance?
	d) Records needed to provide evidence that the realization processes and resulting product meet requirements (see 4.2.4)?
	Is the output of this planning in a form suitable for the organization's method of operations?
	Does the organization establish documented requirements for risk management throughout product realization and are records arising from risk management maintained (see 4.2.4)?

Doc. Reference	Adequate?	Stage I (clauses marked *)	Stage II

	REQUIREMENTS
Brazil	Verify that the manufacturer has established and maintains a continuous process of risk management which covers the entire life cycle of the product. Possible hazards must be identified in both, normal and fault conditions, including those arising from human factors issues. The risk associated with those hazards, shall be calculated. Risks must be analyzed, evaluated and controlled, as necessary. Effectiveness of risk controls implemented shall be evaluated [RDC ANVISA 2001/56 :2013/16, RDC ANVISA :2013/16 2.4].
EU	Does the supplier evaluate the need for risk analysis throughout the design process and maintain records of any risk analysis performed? (MDD Annex 1)

Doc. Reference	Adequate?	Stage I (clauses marked *)	Stage II

	REQUIREMENTS
Brazil	Verify that procedures ensure that the device design is correctly translated into production specifications [RDC ANVISA 4.1.7 :2013/16]. Confirm that the manufacturer ensures that the design release occurs only after the approval(s) of a designated person. Before the final release, design and development records must be reviewed to confirm that the design is complete and that the final design meets the approved design. Final release, including signature(s) (manual or electronic) and dates, shall be documented [RDC ANVISA 4.1.11 ,4.1.9 :2013/16]. Verify that production specifications are documented (e.g. Device Master Record – DMR). The record shall include or make reference to: a) device specifications, including software source code (if applicable), drawings, composition (BOM – bill of materials), etc.; b) production specifications (ex. work instructions, environmental controls, measurement equipment, etc.); c) labeling and packaging specifications; c) measurements, inspections, and tests, with acceptance criteria; and d) methods and procedures for installation and servicing (if applicable) [RDC ANVISA 4.2 :2013/16].

7.2.1 Determination of requirements related to the product	
	Has the organization determined:
	a) Requirements specified by the customer, including the requirements for delivery and post-delivery activities?
	b) Requirements not stated by the customer but necessary for specified or intended use, where known?
	c) Statutory and regulatory requirements related to the product?
	d) Any additional requirements determined by the organization?

Doc. Reference	Adequate?	Stage I (clauses marked *)	Stage II

	REQUIREMENTS
Brazil	Verifiy for domestic and international manufacturers that the products already distributed in the Brazilian market are registered/notified with ANVISA [Brazilian Federal Law n° 76/6360]. • Medical devices registration/notification: Device marketing authorization shall be requested to ANVISA by the domestic manufacturer or importer (legal representative) formally established in Brazil. Registration is a comprehensive process for market authorization, applied to medical devices in classes III and IV, and some class I and II devices, listed on an exception list [ANVISA IN n° 2011/03]. Notification is a simplified market authorization process, applied to medical device classes I and II, not listed on the exception list [ANVISA IN n° 2011/03]. Both registration and notification are valid for 5 years – renewal of these authorizations shall be requested upon time defined at Brazilian Law 1976/6360. • Establishment license: Domestic manufacturer: shall be authorized by ANVISA, at a minimum, as a manufacturer of medical devices. This license includes authorization to store and distribute medical devices. Importer: the importer is considered the legal representative of the international manufacturer in Brazil and shall be authorized by ANVISA to import, store, and distribute medical devices.

Doc. Reference	Adequate?	Stage I (clauses marked *)	Stage II

	REQUIREMENTS
EU	Vefiy that manufacturing maintains files containing or refer to the location of objective evidence establishing the safety and effectiveness of the device as required by Annex 1 of the MDD. Verify that the manufacturer followed a defined and effective process to establish and maintain a file containing documents defining product specifications and quality system requirements for each newa and existing type/modes of medical devices. Since the last audit, has the manufacturer introduced new products in the EU? Has the manufacturer followed a defined and effective process to obtain an approval from the Notified Body to CE mark a product prior to selling it in the EU? (does not apply to class I devices)
7.2.2 Review of requirements related to the product	
	Does the organization review the requirements related to the product?
	Is this review conducted prior to the organization's commitment to supply a product to the customer (e.g. submission of tenders, acceptance of contracts or orders, acceptance of changes to contracts or orders)?
	Does the organization ensure that:
	a) Product requirements are defined and documented?
	b) Contract or order requirements differing from those previously expressed are resolved?
	c) The organization has the ability to meet the defined requirements?
	Are records of the results of the review and actions arising from the review maintained (see 4.2.4)?

Doc. Reference	Adequate?	Stage I (clauses marked *)	Stage II

	REQUIREMENTS
	Where the customer provides no documented statement of requirement, are the customer requirements confirmed by the organization before acceptance?
	Where product requirements are changed, does the organization ensure that relevant documents are amended and that relevant personnel are made aware of the changed requirements?
7.2.3 Customer communication	
	Has the organization determined and implemented effective arrangements for communicating with customers in relation to:
	a) Product information?
	b) Enquiries, contracts or order handling, including amendments?
	c) Customer feedback, including customer complaints? (see 8.2.1)
	d) Advisory notices? (see 8.5.1)
7.3 Design and development	
7.3.1 Design and/or development planning	
	Has the organization established documented procedures for design and development?
	Does the organization plan and control the design and development of product?
	During the design and development planning, does the organization determine:
	a) The design and development stages?
	b) The review, verification, validation and design transfer activities (see Note) that are appropriate at each design and development stage?
	c) The responsibilities and authorities for design and development?

Doc. Reference	Adequate?	Stage I (clauses marked *)	Stage II

	REQUIREMENTS
	Does the organization manage the interfaces between different groups involved in design and development to ensure effective communication and clear assignment of responsibility?
	Is planning output documented, and updated as appropriate, as the design and development progresses? (See 4.2.3)
7.3.2 Design and development inputs	
	Have inputs relating to product requirements been determined and records maintained (see 4.2.4)?
	Do these inputs include:
	a) Functional, performance and safety requirements, according to the intended use?
	b) Applicable statutory and regulatory requirements?
	c) Where applicable, information derived from previous similar designs?
	d) Other requirements essential for design and development?
	e) Output(s) of risk management (see 7.1)?
	Are these inputs reviewed for adequacy and approved?
	Are requirements complete, unambiguous and not in conflict with each other?
7.3.3 Design and development outputs	
	Are the outputs of design and development provided in a form that enables verification against the design and development input, and is it approved prior to release?

Doc. Reference	Adequate?	Stage I (clauses marked *)	Stage II

	REQUIREMENTS
	Do design and development outputs:
	a) meet the input requirements for design and development?
	b) Provide appropriate information for purchasing, production and for service provision?
	c) Contain or reference product acceptance criteria?
	d) Specify the characteristics of the product that are essential for its safe and proper use?
	Are records of the design and development outputs maintained (see 4.2.4)?
7.3.4 Design and development review	
	At suitable stages, are systematic reviews of design and development performed in accordance with planned arrangements (see 7.3.1):
	a) To evaluate the ability of the results of design and development to meet requirements?
	b) To identify any problems and propose necessary actions?
	Do participants in such reviews include representatives of functions concerned with the design and development stage(s) being reviewed, as well as other specialist personnel (see 5.5.1 and 6.2.1)?
	Are records of the results of the reviews and any necessary actions maintained (see 4.2.4)?
EU	Does the supplier evaluate the need for risk analysis throughout the design process and maintain records of any risk analysis performed? (MDD Annex 1)
7.3.5 Design and development verification	
	Is verification performed in accordance with planned arrangements (see 7.3.1) to ensure that the design and development outputs have met the design and development input requirements?
	Are records of the results of the verification and any necessary actions maintained?

Doc. Reference	Adequate?	Stage I (clauses marked *)	Stage II

	REQUIREMENTS	
	7.3.6 Design and development validation	
	Is design and development validation performed in accordance with planned arrangements (see 7.3.1) to ensure that the resulting product is capable of meeting the requirements for the specified application or intended use?	
	Is validation completed prior to the delivery or implementation of the product (see Note 1)?	
	Are records of the results of validation and any necessary actions maintained (see 4.2.4)?	
	As part of design and development validation, does the organization perform clinical evaluations and/or evaluation of performance of the medical device, as required by national or regional regulations (see Note 2)?	
Brazil	Verify that design validation has been performed under defined operating conditions on initial production units, lots, or batches. Validation shall include device testing under real or simulated conditions of use. Design validation shall include software validation, as necessary. Stability studies shall be performed as necessary [RDC ANVISA :2013/16 4.1.8].	
	7.3.7 Control of design and development changes	
	Are design and development changes identified and records maintained?	
	Are changes reviewed, verified, and validated, as appropriate, and approved before implementation?	
	Does the review of design and development changes include evaluation of the effect of the changes on constituent parts and product already delivered?	
	Are records of the results of the review of changes and any necessary actions maintained?	

Doc. Reference	Adequate?	Stage I (clauses marked *)	Stage II

	REQUIREMENTS
Brazil	If the medical device evaluated is already registered/notified with ANVISA, verify that the design change was correctly and promptly submitted to ANVISA for approval, when applicable [Brazilian Law 76/6360 - Art. 13].
EU	Do documented procedures identify the need to report essential changes to the Notified Body, (MDD Annex II, V, VI, 3.4)
7.4 Purchasing	
7.4.1 Purchasing process	
	Has the organization established documented procedures to ensure that purchased product conforms to specified purchase requirements?
	Is the type and extent of control applied to the supplier and the purchased product dependent upon the effect of the purchased product on subsequent product realization or the final product?
	Does the organization evaluate and select suppliers based on their ability to supply product in accordance with the organization's requirements?
	Have criteria for selection, evaluation and re-evaluation been established?
	Are records of the results of evaluation and any necessary actions arising from the evaluation maintained (see 4.2.4)?
Brazil	Confirm that the manufacturer establishes and maintains records of approved suppliers, contractors, and consultants [RDC ANVISA 2.5.3 ,2.3.3 :2013/16].

Doc. Reference	Adequate?	Stage I (clauses marked *)	Stage II

	REQUIREMENTS
7.4.2 Purchasing information	
	Does purchasing information describe the product to be purchased, including where appropriate:
	a) Requirements for approval of product, procedures, processes and equipment?
	b) Requirements for qualification of personnel?
	c) Quality management system requirements?
	Does the organization ensure the adequacy of specified purchase requirements prior to their communication to the supplier?
	To the extent required for traceability given in 7.5.3.2, does the organization maintain relevant purchasing information, i.e. documents (see 4.2.3) and records (see 4.2.4)?
Brazil	Confirm that an agreement is established and documented in which suppliers agree to notify the manufacturer of any change in the product or service, so that the manufacturer can determine whether the change affects the quality of the finished product [RDC ANVISA 2.5.5 :2013/16].
7.4.3 Verification of purchased product	
	Has the organization established and implemented the inspection or other activities necessary for ensuring that purchased product meets specified purchase requirements?
	Where the organization or its customer intends to perform verification at the supplier's premises, does the organization state the intended verification arrangements and method of product release in the purchasing information?
	Are records of the verification maintained (see 4.2.4)?
Brazil	Verify that the manufacturer has established and maintains procedures to ensure the retention of components, raw materials, in-process products and returned products until inspections, tests or other specified verifications have been performed and documented [RDC ANVISA 5.3.3 :2013/16].

Doc. Reference	Adequate?	Stage I (clauses marked *)	Stage II

	REQUIREMENTS

7.5 Production and service provision	
7.5.1 Control of production and service provision	
7.5.1.1 General Requirements	
	Does the organization plan and carry out production and service provision under controlled conditions?
	Do the controlled conditions include, as applicable:
	a) The availability of information that describes the characteristics of the product?
	b) The availability of documented procedures, documented requirements, work instructions, reference materials and reference measurement procedures as necessary?
	c) The use of suitable equipment?
	d) The availability and use of monitoring and measuring devices?
	e) The implementation of monitoring and measurement?
	f) The implementation of release, delivery and post-delivery activities?
	g) The implementation of defined operations for labeling and packaging?
	Does the organization establish and maintain a record (see 4.2.4) for each batch of medical devices that provides traceability to the extent specified in 7.5.3 and identifies the amount manufactured and amount approved for distribution?
	Is the batch record verified and approved?

Doc. Reference	Adequate?	Stage I (clauses marked *)	Stage II

	REQUIREMENTS
Brazil	Determine whether the manufacturer has established and maintained a procedure for change control in order to track changes in auxiliary systems, software, equipment, processes, methods or other changes that may affect the quality of products, including risk assessment within the risk management process. The procedure must describe the actions to be taken, including, when appropriate, the need for re-qualification or re-validation. Verify that changes are formally requested, documented and approved before implementation [RDC ANVISA 5.6.2 ;5.6.1 ;5.6 :2013/16].

7.5.1.2 Control of production and service provision — Specific requirement	
7.5.1.2.1 Cleanliness of product and contamination control	
	Does the organization establish documented requirements for cleanliness of product if:
	a) Product is cleaned by the organization prior to sterilization and/or its use, or
	b) Product is supplied non-sterile to be subjected to a cleaning process prior to sterilization and/or its use, or
	c) Product is supplied to be used non-sterile and its cleanliness is of significance in use, or
	d) Process agents are to be removed from product during manufacture?
	If product is cleaned in accordance with a) or b) above, the requirements contained in 6.4 a) and 6.4 b) do not apply prior to the cleaning process.

Doc. Reference	Adequate?	Stage I (clauses marked *)	Stage II

	REQUIREMENTS
Brazil	Confirm that a pest control program has been established and where chemicals are used as part of the pestcontrol program, the company must ensure that they do not affect product quality [RDC ANVISA 2013:5.1.3.4/16]. Verify that the manufacturer has established and maintains housekeeping procedures and schedules forproduction areas and warehouses, in conformance with production specifications [RDC ANVISA 2013:5.1.3.1/16].
7.5.1.2.2 Installation activities	
	If appropriate, does the organization establish documented requirements which contain acceptance criteria for installing and verifying the installation of the medical device?
	If the agreed customer requirements allow installation to be performed other than by the organization or its authorized agent, does the organization provide documented requirements for installation and verification?
	Are records of installation and verification performed by the organization or its authorized agent maintained (see 4.2.4)?
7.5.1.2.3 Servicing activities	
	If servicing is a specified requirement, does the organization establish documented procedures, work instructions and reference materials and reference measurement procedures, as necessary, for performing servicing activities and verifying that they meet the specified requirements?
	Are records of servicing activities carried out by the organization maintained (see 4.2.4)?

Doc. Reference	Adequate?	Stage I (clauses marked *)	Stage II
		*	

	REQUIREMENTS
Brazil	Confirm that the manufacturer has established and maintains procedures to ensure that records of servicing activities are kept with the following information: the product serviced; the control number of product serviced; the date of completion of service; identification of the service provider; description of service performed; and results of inspections and tests performed [RDC ANVISA :2013/16 8.2.1]. Verify that the manufacturer periodically reviews the records of servicing activities. In cases where the analysis identifies trends that pose danger or records involving death or serious injury, a corrective or preventive action must be initiated [RDC ANVISA 8.2.2 :2013/16].
7.5.1.3 Particular requirements for sterile medical devices	
	Does the organization maintain records of the process parameters for the sterilization process which was used for each sterilization batch (see 4.2.4)?
	Are sterilization records traceable to each production batch of medical devices (see 7.5.1.1)?
7.5.2 Validation of processes for production and service provision	
7.5.2.1 General requirements	
	Does the organization validate any processes for production and service provision where the resulting output cannot be verified by subsequent monitoring or measurement? (this includes any processes where deficiencies become apparent only after the product is in use or the service has been delivered)
	Does validation demonstrate the ability of the processes to achieve planned results?

Doc. Reference	Adequate?	Stage I (clauses marked *)	Stage II

	REQUIREMENTS
	Has the organization established arrangements for these processes including, as applicable:
	a) Defined criteria for review and approval of the processes?
	b) Approval of equipment and qualification of personnel?
	c) Use of specific methods and procedures?
	d) Requirements for records (see 4.2.4)?
	e) Re-validation?
	Has the organization established documented procedures for the validation of the application of computer software (and changes to such software and/or its application) for production and service provision that affect the ability of the product to conform to specified requirements?
	Are such software applications validated prior to initial use?
	Are records of validation maintained (see 4.2.4)?
Brazil	Verify that analytical methods, utilities, computer systems and automated software that can adversely affect product quality or the quality system are validated, periodically reviewed and, when necessary, revalidated[RDC ANVISA 5.5.3 ,5.5.2 :2013/16].
Brazil	Verify that processes requiring validation are validated according to previously established protocols. The results of validations, including date and identification of the person responsible for its approval, must be recorded [RDC ANVISA 5.5.1 :2013/16].
7.5.2.2 Particular requirements for sterile medical devices	
	Has the organization established documented procedures for the validation of sterilization processes?
	Are sterilization processes validated prior to initial use?
	Are records of validation of each sterilization process maintained (see 4.2.4)?

Doc. Reference	Adequate?	Stage I (clauses marked *)	Stage II

	REQUIREMENTS

7.5.3 Identification and traceability	

7.5.3.1 Identification	
	Does the organization identify the product by suitable means throughout product realization and does the organization establish documented procedures for such product identification?
	Has the organization established documented procedures to ensure that medical devices returned to the organization are identified and distinguished from conforming product [see 6.4 d)]?

7.5.3.2 Traceability	

7.5.3.2.1 General	
	Has the organization established documented procedures for traceability?
	Do such procedures define the extent of product traceability and the records required (see 8.3 ,4.2.4 and 8.5)?
	Does the organization control and record the unique identification of the product, where traceability is a requirement (see 4.2.4)?
Brazil	Verify that the manufacturer has established and maintains procedures to ensure integrity and to prevent accidental mixing of labels, instructions, and packaging materials [RDC ANVISA 5.2.2.1 :2013/16]. Confirm that the manufacturer has ensured that labels are designed, printed and, where applicable, applied so that they remain legible and attached to the product during processing, storage, handling and use [RDC ANVISA 5.2.2.2 :2013/16].
US	If a control number is required for traceability, confirm that such control number is on or accompanies the device throughout distribution [21 CFR 820.120(e)].

Doc. Reference	Adequate?	Stage I (clauses marked *)	Stage II

	REQUIREMENTS
EU	Does the manufacturer have procedures identifying the requirements of labeling and instructions for use as defined in MDD, Annex 1 point 13, and is regulations for CE marking included in these procedures. (MDD 3, Article 17 and Annex 12).
	Are language requirements defined in procedures for the information identified in MDD, Annex 1point 13 for the applicable markets.
7.5.3.2.2 Particular requirements for active implantable medical devices and	
	In defining the records required for traceability, does the organization include records of all components, materials and work environment conditions, if these could cause the medical device not to satisfy its specified requirements?
	Does the organization require that its agents or distributors maintain records of the distribution of medical devices to allow traceability and that such records be available for inspection?
	Are records of the name and address of the shipping package consignee maintained (see 4.2.4)?
7.5.3.3 Status identification	
	Does the organization identify the product status with respect to monitoring and measurement requirements?
	Is the identification of product status maintained throughout production, storage, installation and servicing of the product to ensure that only product that has passed the required inspections and tests (or released under an authorized concession) is dispatched, used or installed?
7.5.4 Customer property	
	Does the organization exercise care with customer property while it is under the organization's control or being used by the organization?

Doc. Reference	Adequate?	Stage I (clauses marked *)	Stage II

e medical devices

	REQUIREMENTS
	Does the organization identify, verify, protect and safeguard customer property provided for use or incorporation into the product?
	If any customer property is lost, damaged, or otherwise found to be unsuitable for use, is this reported to the customer and are records maintained (see 4.2.4)?
7.5.5 Preservation of product	
	Has the organization established documented procedures or documented work instructions for preserving the conformity of product during internal processing and delivery to the intended destination?
	Does this preservation include identification, handling, packaging, storage and protection, and also apply to the constituent parts of a product?
	Has the organization established documented procedures or documented work instructions for the control of product with a limited shelf-life or requiring special storage conditions?
	Are such special storage conditions controlled and recorded (see 4.2.4)?
Brazil	Verify that the manufacturer has established procedures for the packaging of products in order to protect the product from deterioration, damage, or contamination during processing, storage, handling, and distribution [RDC ANVISA 5.2.1 :2013/16].
7.6 Control of monitoring and measuring devices	
	Does the organization determine monitoring and measuring to be undertaken and the monitoring and measuring devices needed to provide evidence of conformity of product to determined requirements (guide reference 7.2.1)?

Doc. Reference	Adequate?	Stage I (clauses marked *)	Stage II

	REQUIREMENTS
	Has the organization established documented procedures to ensure that monitoring and measurement can be carried out and are carried out in a manner that is consistent with the monitoring and measurement requirements?
	Where necessary to ensure valid results, is measuring equipment:
	a) Calibrated or verified at specified intervals, or prior to use, against measurement standards traceable to international or national measurement standards; where no such standards exist, is the basis used for calibration or verification recorded?
	b) Adjusted or re-adjusted as necessary?
	c) Identified to enable the calibration status to be determined?
	d) Safeguarded from adjustments that would invalidate the measurement result?
	e) Protected from damage and deterioration during handling, maintenance and storage?
	Does the organization assess and record the validity of the previous measuring results when the equipment is found not to conform to requirements?
	Does the organization take appropriate action on the equipment and any product affected?
	Are records of the results of calibration and verification maintained (see 4.2.4)?
	When used in the monitoring and measurement of specified requirements, is the ability of computer software to satisfy the intended application confirmed prior to initial use and reconfirmed as necessary ?

Doc. Reference	Adequate?	Stage I (clauses marked *)	Stage II

	REQUIREMENTS

8 Measurement, analysis and improvement	
8.1 General	
	Does the organization plan and implement the monitoring, measurement, analysis and improvement processes needed:
	a) To demonstrate conformity of the product?
	b) To ensure conformity of the quality management system?
	c) To maintain the effectiveness of the quality management system?
	Does this include determination of applicable methods, including statistical techniques, and the extent of their use?
Brazil	Verify that the organization has established and maintained procedures for identifying valid statistical techniques required for verifying the quality system performance and process capability for achieving established specifications [RDC ANVISA 9.1 :2013/16].
8.2 Monitoring and measurement	
8.2.1 Feedback	
	As one of the measurements of the performance of the quality management system, does the organization monitor information relating to whether the organization has met customer requirements?
	Have the methods for obtaining and using this information been determined?
	Has the organization established a documented procedure for a feedback system [see 7.2.3 c)] to provide early warning of quality problems and for input into the corrective and preventive action processes (see 8.5.2 and 8.5.3)?
	If national or regional regulations require the organization to gain experience from the post-production phase, does the review of this experience form part of the feedback system (see 8.5.1)?

Doc. Reference	Adequate?	Stage I (clauses marked *)	Stage II

	REQUIREMENTS
Brazil	Verify that each manufacturer has established and maintains procedures to receive, examine, evaluate, investigate and document complaints. Such procedures must ensure that: (1) Complaints are received, documented, analyzed, evaluated, investigated and documented by a formally designated unit; (2) Where applicable, complaints must be reported to the competent health authority; (3) Complaints must be examined to determine whether an investigation is necessary. When an investigation is not done, the unit must maintain a record that includes the reason that the investigation was not performed and the name of the responsible for that decision; (4) Each manufacturer must examine, evaluate and investigate all complaints involving possible nonconformities of the product. Any claim for death, injury or threat to public health must be immediately reviewed, evaluated and investigated. (5) The records of the investigation must include: Product name; Date of receipt of the complaint; Any control number used; Name, address and telephone number of the complainant; Nature of complaint; and Data and research results including actions taken [RDC ANVISA 7.2 :2013/16].
8.2.2 Internal audit	

Doc. Reference	Adequate?	Stage I (clauses marked *)	Stage II

	REQUIREMENTS
	Does the organization conduct internal audits at planned intervals to determine whether the quality management system
	a) Conforms to the planned arrangements (see 7.1), to the requirements of this International Standard and to the quality management system requirements established by the organization?
	b) Is effectively implemented and maintained?
	Is an audit programme planned, taking into consideration the status and importance of the processes and areas to be audited, as well as the results of previous audits?
	Are the audit criteria, scope, frequency and methods defined?
	Does selection of auditors and conduct of audits ensure objectivity and impartiality of the audit process (e.g. auditors shall not audit their own work)?
	Are the responsibilities and requirements for planning and conducting audits, and for reporting results and maintaining records (see 4.2.4) defined in a documented procedure?
	Does management responsible for the area being audited ensure that actions are taken without undue delay to eliminate detected nonconformities and their causes?
	Do follow-up activities include the verification of the actions taken and the reporting of verification results? (see 8.5.2)
Brazil	Verify that quality audits are conducted by trained people in accordance with established audit procedures [RDC ANVISA 7.3.2 :2013/16].
8.2.3 Measurement and monitoring of processes	
	Does the organization apply suitable methods for monitoring and, where applicable, measurement of the quality management system processes?

Doc. Reference	Adequate?	Stage I (clauses marked *)	Stage II

	REQUIREMENTS
	Do these methods demonstrate the ability of the processes to achieve planned results?
	When planned results are not achieved, is correction and corrective action taken, as appropriate, to ensure conformity of the product?
Brazil	Verify that processes which cannot be fully verified are conducted in accordance with established procedures and parameters to ensure conformance to specifications. Critical parameters should be monitored and recorded in the batch record [RDC ANVISA 5.1.6 :2013/16].
8.2.4 Monitoring and measurement of product	
8.2.4.1 General requirements	
	Does the organization monitor and measure the characteristics of the product to verify that product requirements have been met?
	Is this carried out at appropriate stages of the product realization process in accordance with the planned arrangements (see 7.1) and documented procedures (see 7.5.1.1)?
	Is evidence of conformity with the acceptance criteria maintained?
	Do records indicate the person(s) authorizing release of the product (see 4.2.4)?
	Does the organization ensure that product release and service delivery do not proceed until the planned arrangements (see 7.1) have been satisfactorily completed?

Doc. Reference	Adequate?	Stage I (clauses marked *)	Stage II

	REQUIREMENTS
Brazil	Verify that the device history record of the product includes or refers to the following information: date of manufacture; components used; quantity manufactured; results of inspections and tests; parameters of special processes; quantity released for distribution; labeling; identification of the serial number or batch of production; and final release of the product [RDC ANVISA 3.2.1 :2013/16]. Verify that labeling has not been released for storage or use until a designated individual has examined the labeling for accuracy. The approval, including date, name, and physical or electronic signature of the person responsible, must be documented in the device history record [RDC ANVISA 5.2.2.3 :2013/16].
Brazil	Verify that sampling plans are defined and based on valid statistical rationale. Each manufacturer must establish and maintain procedures to ensure that sampling methods are suitable for their intended use and are reviewed regularly. A review of sampling plans should consider the occurrence of nonconforming product, quality audit reports, complaints and other indicators [RDC ANVISA 9.2 :2013/16].
8.2.4.2 Particular requirement for active implantable medical devices and in	
	Does the organization record (see 4.2.4) the identity of personnel performing any inspection or testing?
8.3 Control of nonconforming product	
	Does the organization ensure that product which does not conform to product requirements is identified and controlled to prevent its unintended use or delivery?
	Are the controls and related responsibilities and authorities for dealing with nonconforming product defined in a documented procedure?

Doc. Reference	Adequate?	Stage I (clauses marked *)	Stage II
medical devices			

	REQUIREMENTS
	Does the organization deal with nonconforming product by one or more of the following ways?
	a) By taking action to eliminate the detected nonconformity
	b) By authorizing its use, release or acceptance under concession
	c) By taking action to preclude its original intended use or application
	Does the organization ensure that nonconforming product is accepted by concession only if regulatory requirements are met?
	Are records of the identity of the person(s) authorizing the concession maintained (see 4.2.4)?
	Are records of the nature of nonconformities and any subsequent actions taken, including concessions obtained maintained (see 4.2.4)?
	When nonconforming product is corrected, is it subject to re-verification to demonstrate conformity to the requirements?
	When nonconforming product is detected after delivery or use has started, does the organization take action appropriate to the effects, or potential effects, of the nonconformity?
	If product needs to be reworked (one or more times), does the organization document the rework process in a work instruction that has undergone the same authorization and approval procedure as the original work instruction?
	Prior to authorization and approval of the work instruction, is a determination of any adverse effect of the rework upon product made and documented (see 4.2.3 and 7.5.1)?

Doc. Reference	Adequate?	Stage I (clauses marked *)	Stage II

	REQUIREMENTS
Brazil	Confirm that the evaluation of non-conforming product includes a determination of the need for an investigation and notification of the persons or organizations responsible for the nonconformance. The evaluation and any investigation must be documented [RDC ANVISA 6.5.1 :2013/16].
Brazil	Verify that the manufacturer has procedures to determine the product recall and other field actions that are relevant in the case of products already distributed [RDC ANVISA 7.1.1.8 :2013/16].
8.4 Analysis of data	
	Does the organization establish documented procedures to determine, collect and analyse appropriate data to demonstrate the suitability and effectiveness of the quality management system and to evaluate if improvement of the effectiveness of the quality management system can be made?
	Does this include data generated as a result of monitoring and measurement and from other relevant sources?
	Does the analysis of data provide information relating to:
	a) Feedback (see 8.2.1)?
	b) Conformity to product requirements? (See 7.2.1)
	c) Characteristics and trends of processes and products including opportunities for preventive action?
	d) Suppliers?
	Are records of the results of the analysis of data maintained (see 4.2.4)?
8.5 Improvement	
8.5.1 General	

Doc. Reference	Adequate?	Stage I (clauses marked *)	Stage II

	REQUIREMENTS
	Does the organization identify and implement any changes necessary to ensure and maintain the continued suitability and effectiveness of the quality management system through the use of the quality policy, quality objectives, audit results, analysis of data, corrective and preventive actions and management review?
	Does the organization establish documented procedures for the issue and implementation of advisory notices and are these procedures capable of being implemented at any time?
Brazil	Verify that procedures and work flows were established in order to identify when field actions (recalls and corrections) are necessary, in accordance with the organization's post-market surveillance system and quality system. [RDC ANVISA 2009/67 RDC ANVISA 2012/23 RDC ANVISA 7.1.1.8 :2013/16]
EU	Are the procedures for Vigilance reporting in conformance with MDD Annex II, V, and VI (MEDDEV 1-2.12)
	Are records of all customer complaint investigations maintained (see 4.2.4)?
	If investigation determines that the activities outside the organization contributed to the customer complaint, is relevant information exchanged between the organizations involved (see 4.1)?
	If any customer complaint is not followed by corrective and/or preventive action, is the reason authorized (see 5.5.1) and recorded (see 4.2.4)?

Doc. Reference	Adequate?	Stage I (clauses marked *)	Stage II

	REQUIREMENTS
Brazil	Verify that the manufacturer has ensured that information about quality problems or nonconforming products are properly disseminated to those directly involved in the maintenance of product quality and to prevent occurrence of such problems [RDC ANVISA 7.1.1.6 :2013/16].
	If national or regional regulations require notification of adverse events that meet specific reporting criteria, does the organization establish documented procedures to such notification to regulatory authorities?
Brazil	Verify that a post-market surveillance system is established and implemented in the organization and integrated into the Quality System, with procedures and work flows established to ensure the correct and the prompt identification of adverse events, the performance of investigations and use of the results to improve the safety and effectiveness of the device when necessary [RDC ANVISA 2009/67 RDC ANVISA 7.1.1.7 :2013/16]
EU	Are procedures for the reporting of recall to the relevant competent authority and the NB compliant? (MDD, Annex II, V, VI, 3.1)
8.5.2 Corrective action	
	Does the organization take action to eliminate the cause of nonconformities in order to prevent recurrence and are corrective actions appropriate to the effects of the nonconformities encountered?

Doc. Reference	Adequate?	Stage I (clauses marked *)	Stage II

	REQUIREMENTS	
	Has a documented procedure been established to define requirements for:	
	a) Reviewing nonconformities (including customer complaints)?	
	b) Determining the causes of nonconformities?	
	c) Evaluating the need for action to ensure that nonconformities do no recur?	
	d) Determining and implementing action needed, including, if appropriate, updating documentation (see 4.2)?	
	e) Recording of the results of any investigation and of action taken (see 4.2.4)?	
	f) Reviewing the corrective action taken and its effectiveness?	
8.5.3 Preventive action		
	Does the organization determine action to eliminate the causes of potential nonconformities in order to prevent their occurrence and are preventive actions appropriate to the effects of the potential problems?	
	Has a documented procedure been established to define requirements for:	
	a) Determining potential nonconformities and their causes?	
	b) Evaluating the need for action to prevent occurrence of nonconformities?	
	c) Determining and implementing action needed?	
	d) Recording of the results of any investigations and of action taken (see 4.2.4)?	
	e) Reviewing preventive action taken and its effectiveness?	

Doc. Reference	Adequate?	Stage I (clauses marked *)	Stage II

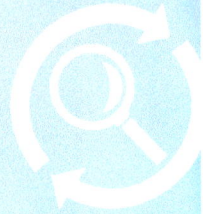

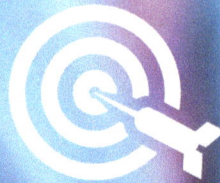

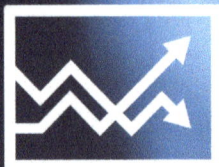

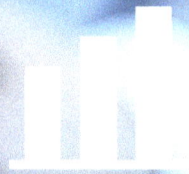

MDSAP
ISO 13485 Requirements &

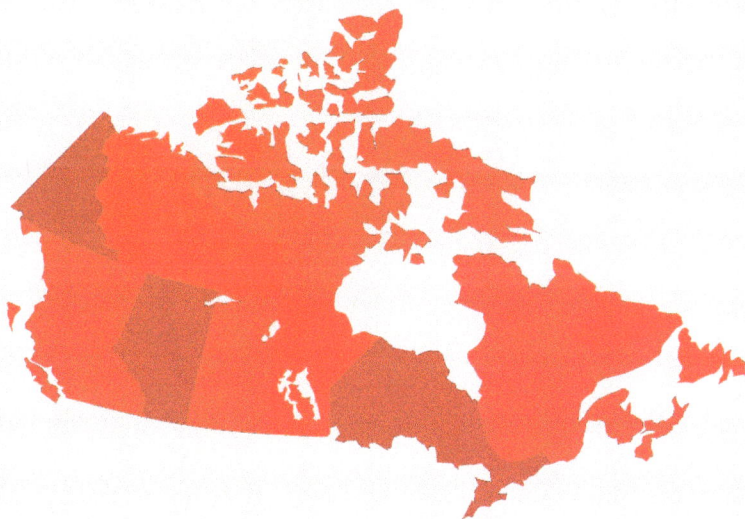

CANADA

Management

The intent of the Management Process is to provide adequate resources for device design, manufacturing, quality assurance, distribution, installation, and servicing activities; to assure the quality management system is functioning properly and effectively; and to monitor the quality management system and make necessary adjustments. A quality management system that has been implemented effectively and is monitored to identify and address existing and potential problems is more likely to produce medical devices that function as intended.

The management representative is responsible for ensuring that the requirements of the quality management system have been effectively defined, documented, implemented, and maintained. Prior to the audit of a process, it may be helpful to interview the management representative (or designee) to obtain an overview of the process and a feel for management's knowledge and understanding of the process.

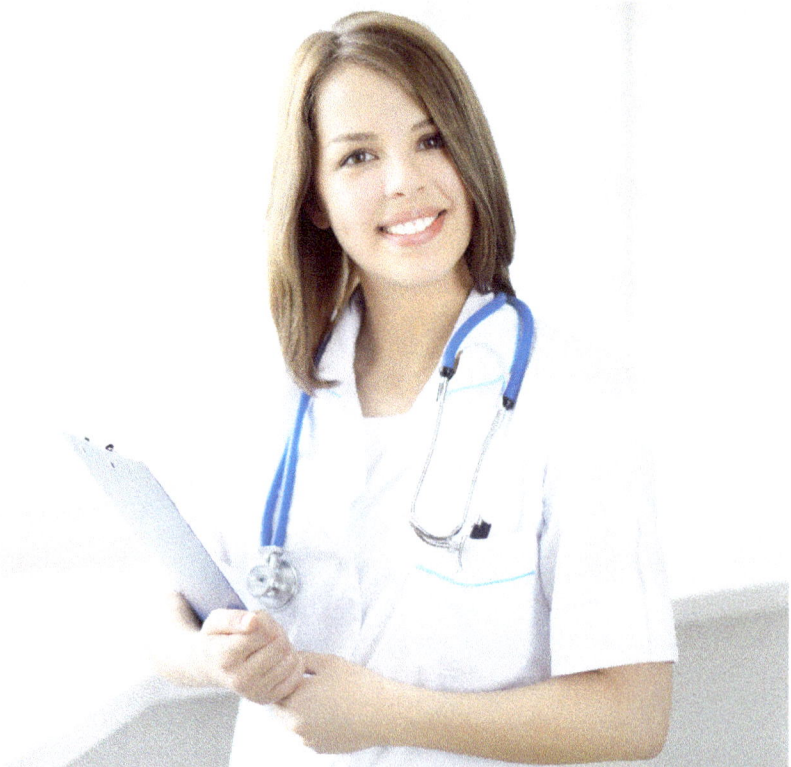

Clause and Regulation:
ISO 13485:2016: 4.1.1, 4.1.2, 4.1.3, 4.2.2, 4.1.4, 5.4.2;
Health Canada Medical Devices Regulations
(SOR /98-282)
FDA: 21 CFR 820.20

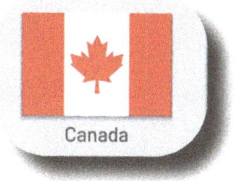
Canada

Verify that the roles and responsibilities of any regulatory correspondents, importers, distributors, or providers of a service are clearly documented in the medical device organization's quality management system and are qualified as suppliers and controlled, as appropriate.

During the audit of the other MDSAP processes, the audit team will have the opportunity to assess whether management is appropriately carrying out its responsibilities; whether the quality policy is understood, implemented, and maintained at all levels of the medical device organization; if the necessary resources are being provided to maintain an effective quality management system; if the management representative has the necessary responsibilities and authorities; the adequacy of the organizational structure; and whether management reviews and quality audits are effective, etc.

Remember that a quality management system that has been implemented effectively, monitored to identify and address existing and potential problems, and has an integrated risk management process utilizing risk-based decision-making is more likely to produce medical devices that function as intended.

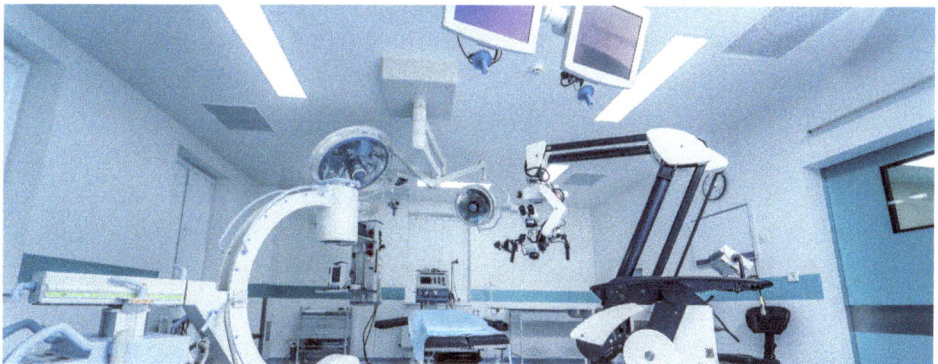

Device Marketing Authorization and Facility Registration

The Device Marketing Authorization and Facility Registration process may be audited as a linkage from the Management process and/or the Design and Development process.

ISO: ISO 13485:2016: 4.1.1, 4.2.1, 5.2, 7.2.1, 7.2.3
Health Canada Medical Devices Regulations
(SOR /98-282)

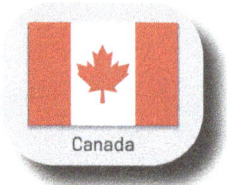

Manufacturer means a person who sells a medical device under their own name, or under a trade-mark, design, trade name or other name or mark owned or controlled by the person, and who is responsible for designing, manufacturing, assembling, processing, labeling, packaging, refurbishing or modifying the device, or for assigning to it a purpose, whether those tasks are performed by that person or on their behalf [CMDR 1].

No person shall import or sell a Class II, III or IV medical device unless the manufacturer of the device holds a license in respect of that device or, if the medical device has been subjected to a change described in section 34, an amended medical device license [CMDR 26]. An application for a medical device license shall be submitted to the Minister by the manufacturer of the medical device in a format established by the Minister
 [CMDR 32].

An application for a medical device license shall include a copy of a quality management system certificate certifying that the quality management system under which the medical device is manufactured (class II) or designed and manufacturer (class III or IV) satisfies National Standard of Canada CAN/CSA-ISO 13485:2016.
[CMDR 32(2)(f); 32(3)(j); 32(4)(p)].

No person shall import or sell a Class II, III or IV medical device unless the Manufacturer of the device holds a license in respect of that device or, if the medical device has been subjected to a change described in section 34 - an amended medical device license
[CMDR 26].

If the Manufacturer proposes to make one or more changes, the Manufacturer shall submit to the Minister, in a format established by the Minister, an application for a medical device license amendment including the information and documents set out in section 32 that are relevant to the change
[CMDR 34].

Every Manufacturer of a licensed medical device shall, annually before November 1 and in a form authorized by the Minister, furnish the Minister with a statement signed by the Manufacturer or by a person authorized to sign on the Manufacturer's behalf describing any change to the information and documents supplied by the Manufacturer with respect to the device, other than those to be submitted under section 34 or 43.1
[CMDR 43].

If the holder of a medical device license discontinues the sale of the medical device in Canada, the licensee shall inform the Minister within 30 days after the discontinuance, and the license shall be cancelled at the time that the Minister is informed
[CMDR 43(3)].

Subject to section 34, if a new or modified quality management system certificate is issued in respect of a licensed medical device, the Manufacturer of the device shall submit a copy of the certificate to the Minister within 30 days after it is issued
[CMDR 43.1].

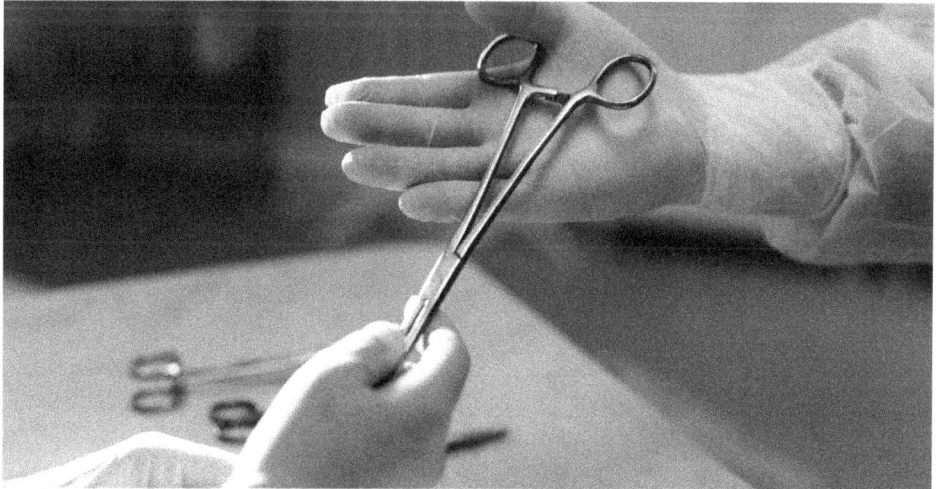

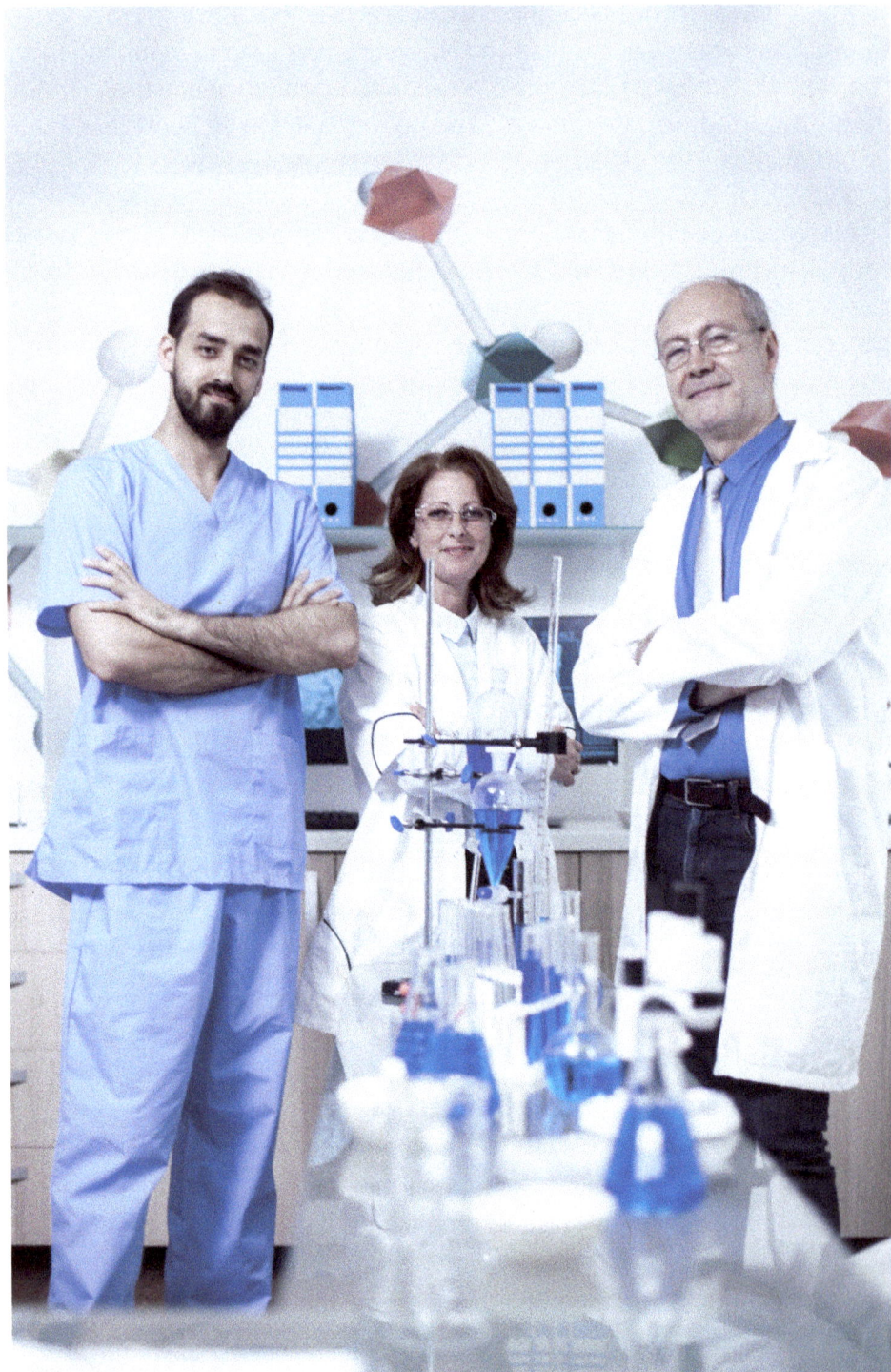

Measurement, Analysis and Improvement

One of the most important activities in the quality management system is the identification of existing and potential causes of product and quality problems. Such causes must be identified so that appropriate and effective corrective or preventive actions can take place. These activities are carried out under the Measurement, Analysis and Improvement process.

Clause and Regulation
ISO: ISO 13485:2016: 4.2.1, 8.1, 8.2.1, 8.2.6, 8.5
HC: CMDR 57-58
HC: CMDR 59-61.1
HC: CMDR 63-65.1

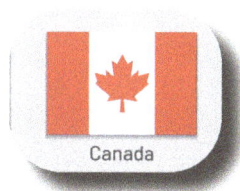
Canada

Verify that the Manufacturer has a process or procedure for identifying a "significant change" to a class III or IV device. Verify that information about "significant changes" is submitted in a medical device license amendment application
[CMDR 1, 34].

Verify that the Manufacturer maintains records of reported problems related to the performance characteristics or safety of a device, including any consumer complaints received by the Manufacturer after the device was first sold in Canada, and all actions taken by the Manufacturer in response to the problems referred to in the complaints .
[CMDR Section 57].

Verify that the Manufacturer has established and implemented documented procedures that will enable it to carry out an effective and timely investigation of the problem reports through the customer complaints, and to carry out an effective and timely recall of the device
[CMDR Section 58].

Medical Device Adverse Events and Advisory Notices Reporting
The Medical Device Adverse Events and Advisory Notices Reporting
process may be audited as a linkage from the Measurement, Analysis
and Improvement process.

Clause and Regulation
ISO: ISO 13485:2016: 4.2.1, 7.2.3, 8.2.2, 8.2.3, 8.3.3
SOR/98-282, Section 59-61.1
SOR/98-282, Section 63 – 65.1

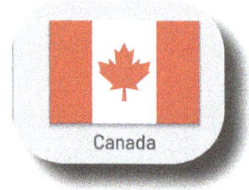

Medical Device Regulations SOR/98-282, Section 59-61.1
Verify that the Manufacturer and the importer of a medical device
make a preliminary and final report to the minister concerning any
incident occurring inside or outside Canada involving a device sold
in Canada:
- Related to the failure of the device or deterioration in its effectiveness or any inadequacy in its labeling or in its directions for use.
- Has led to death or serious deterioration in the state of health of
a patient, user, or other person, or could do so if it were to occur
[CMDR 59].
Verify that the Manufacturer or other person becoming aware of an
event that led to the death or serious deterioration in the state of
health of a patient, a user, or other person provides information in
a preliminary report within 10 days after the person becomes aware
of the event or occurrence [CMDR 60 (1) (a) (i)].
Verify that the Manufacturer or other person becoming aware of an
event that the recurrence of which might lead to the death or serious deterioration in the state of health of a patient, a user, or other
person provides information in a preliminary report within 30 days
after the person becomes aware of the event or occurrence [CMDR
60 (1) (a) (ii)].
Note: The requirement to report incidents meeting the requirements of section 59.(1) that occur outside of Canada does not apply
unless the Manufacturer has indicated, to a regulatory agency of the
country in which the incident occurred, the Manufacturer's intention to take corrective action, or unless the regulatory agency has
required the Manufacturer to take corrective action. [CMDR 59.(2)]
Verify that Manufacturer has made effective arrangements to sub-

mit preliminary reports to the Minister and that the reports contain [CMDR 60 (2)]:

- the identifier of any medical device that is part of a system, test kit, medical device group, medical device family or medical device group family
- if the report is made by:
- the Manufacturer: the name and address of that Manufacturer and of any known importer, and the name, title and telephone and facsimile numbers of a representative of the Manufacturer to contact for any information concerning the incident, or
- the importer of the device: the name and address of the importer and of the Manufacturer, and the name, title and telephone and facsimile numbers of a representative of the importer to contact for any information concerning the incident.
- the date on which the incident came to the attention of the Manufacturer or importer
the details known in respect of the incident, including the date on which the incident occurred and the consequences for the patient, user or other person
- the name, address and telephone number, if known, of the person who reported the incident to the Manufacturer or importer
- the identity of any other medical devices or accessories involved in the incident, if known
- the Manufacturer's or importer's preliminary comments with respect to the incident
- the course of action, including an investigation, that the Manufacturer or importer proposes to follow in respect of the incident and a timetable for carrying out any proposed action and for submitting a final report
- a statement indicating whether a previous report has been made to the Minister with respect to the device and, if so, the date of the report.

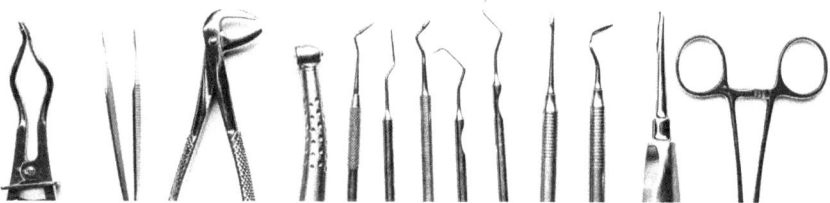

If a preliminary report required by section 60 is submitted to the Minister and/or Importer, verify that the Manufacturer has submitted a final report to the Minister in writing in accordance with the timetable established under CMDR 60(2)(h) and the final report contains [CMDR 61(1)]:

- a description of the incident, including the number of persons who have experienced a serious deterioration in the state of their health or who have died
- a detailed explanation of the cause of the incident and a justification for the actions taken in respect of the incident
- any actions taken as a result of the investigation, which may include:
- increased post-market surveillance of the device
- corrective and preventive action respecting the design and manufacture of the device, and recall of the device.

If the reports required by section 60 and 61 are submitted to the Minister just by the Importer, verify that the Manufacturer has advised the Minister in writing that the reports the Manufacturer and importer would have submitted were identical and that the Manufacturer has permitted the importer to prepare and submit reports to the Minister on the Manufacturer's behalf [CMDR 61.1].

Verify that the Manufacturer and the importer of a medical device, on or before undertaking a recall of a device provide the minister with the following information [CMDR 64]:

- the name of the device and its identifier, including the identifier of any medical device that is part of a system, test kit, medical device group, medical device family or medical device group family
- the name and address of the Manufacturer and importer, and the name and address of the establishment where the device was manufactured, if different from that of the Manufacturer
- the reason for the recall, the nature of the defectiveness or possible defectiveness and the date on and circumstances under which the defectiveness or possible defectiveness was discovered
- an evaluation of the risk associated with the defectiveness or possible defectiveness
- the number of affected units of the device that the Manufacturer or importer:
- manufactured in Canada,

- imported into Canada,
- sold in Canada.
- the period during which the affected units of the device were distributed in Canada by the Manufacturer or importer
- the name of each person to whom the affected device was sold by the Manufacturer or importer and the number of units of the device sold to each person
- a copy of any communication issued with respect to the recall
- the proposed strategy for conducting the recall, including the date for beginning the recall, information as to how and when the Minister will be informed of the progress of the recall and the proposed date for its completion
- the proposed action to prevent a recurrence of the problem
- the name, title and telephone number of the representative of the Manufacturer or importer to contact for any information concerning the recall.

Verify that as soon as possible after the completion of the recall the Manufacturer and the importer reports to the minister the results of the recall and the action taken to prevent a recurrence of the problem [CMDR 65]. If the reports required by section 64 and 65 are submitted to the Minister just by the Importer, verify that the Manufacturer has advised the Minister in writing that the reports the Manufacturer and importer would have submitted were identical and that the Manufacturer has permitted the importer to prepare and submit reports to the Minister on the Manufacturer's behalf [CMDR 65.1].

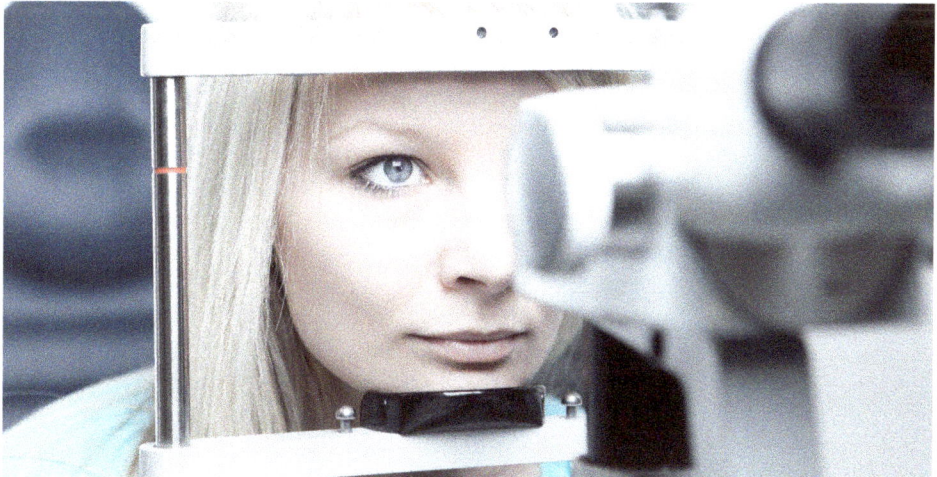

Design and Development

The purpose of the Design and Development process is to control the design of a medical device and to assure that the device meets user needs, intended use, and its specified requirements. Attention to design and development planning, identifying design inputs, developing design outputs, verifying that design outputs meet design inputs, validating the design, controlling design changes, reviewing design results, transferring the design to production, and compiling the appropriate records will help a medical device organization assure that resulting designs will meet user needs, intended uses, and requirements. Review of the Design and Development process will also provide an opportunity to evaluate how the medical device organization has utilized risk management activities to ensure design inputs are comprehensive and meet user needs, to confirm that risk control measures that were planned have been implemented in the design, and to verify that risk control measures are effective in controlling or reducing risk.

Clause and Regulation
ISO: ISO 13485:2016: 4.1.1, 4.2.1, 7.1, 7.3.10, 7.3.2
HC CMDR 9, 10 to 20, 32, 21-23, 66-68

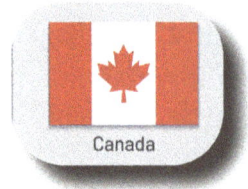

With respect to Class II devices that are not subject to Design and Development controls, verify that the manufacturer has objective evidence to establish that Class II devices meet the safety and effectiveness requirements of section 10 to 20
[CMDR 9, 10 to 20].

Verify that Manufacturers of Class IV devices maintain a quality plan that sets out the specific quality practices, resources, and sequence of activities relevant to the device
[CMDR 32].

Production and Service Controls

The purpose of the Production and Service Controls process is to manufacture products that meet specifications. Developing processes that are adequate to produce devices that meet specifications, validating (or fully verifying the results of) those processes, and monitoring and controlling those processes are all steps that help assure the result will be devices that meet specified requirements. After completing the audit of the medical device organization's Production and Service Controls process, the audit team will return to the Management process to make a final decision of whether top management ensures that an adequate and effective quality management system has been established and maintained at the medical device organization.

Clause and Regulation
ISO: ISO 13485:2016: 7.1, 7.2.1, 7.5.1, 8.2.5, 8.2.6
HC: CMDR 9(2), 14, 17, 21-23, 52-56, 66-68

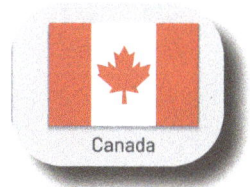

Verify that the Manufacturer maintains objective evidence that devices meet the safety and effectiveness requirements.
[CMDR 9(2)].
Verify that devices sold in Canada have labeling that conforms to Canadian English and French language requirements and contains the Manufacturer's name and address, device identifier, control number (for Class III and IV devices), contents of packaging, sterility, expiry, intended use, directions for use and any special storage conditions [CMDR 21-23].
Verify that the Manufacturer maintains distribution records in respect of a device that will permit a complete and rapid withdrawal of the device from the market [CMDR 52-56].
Verify that the Manufacturer has identified Schedule 2 implants and provides implant registration cards with devices or employs another suitable system approved by Health Canada [CMDR 66-68].
Verify that the Manufacturer of devices that are listed on Schedule 2 of the Medical Devices Regulations maintains distribution records of these devices as well as any information received on implant registration cards related to these Schedule 2 devices [CMDR 54].

Reviewing a validation

During review of a validation study, determine when applicable whether:

- The instruments used to generate the data were properly calibrated and maintained
- Predetermined product and process specifications were established
- Sampling plans used to collect test samples are based on a statistically valid rationale
- Data demonstrates predetermined specifications were met consistently
- Process tolerance limits were challenged
- Process equipment was properly installed, adjusted, and maintained
- Process monitoring instruments were properly calibrated and maintained
- Changes to the validated process were appropriately challenged (if applicable)
- Process operators were appropriately qualified.

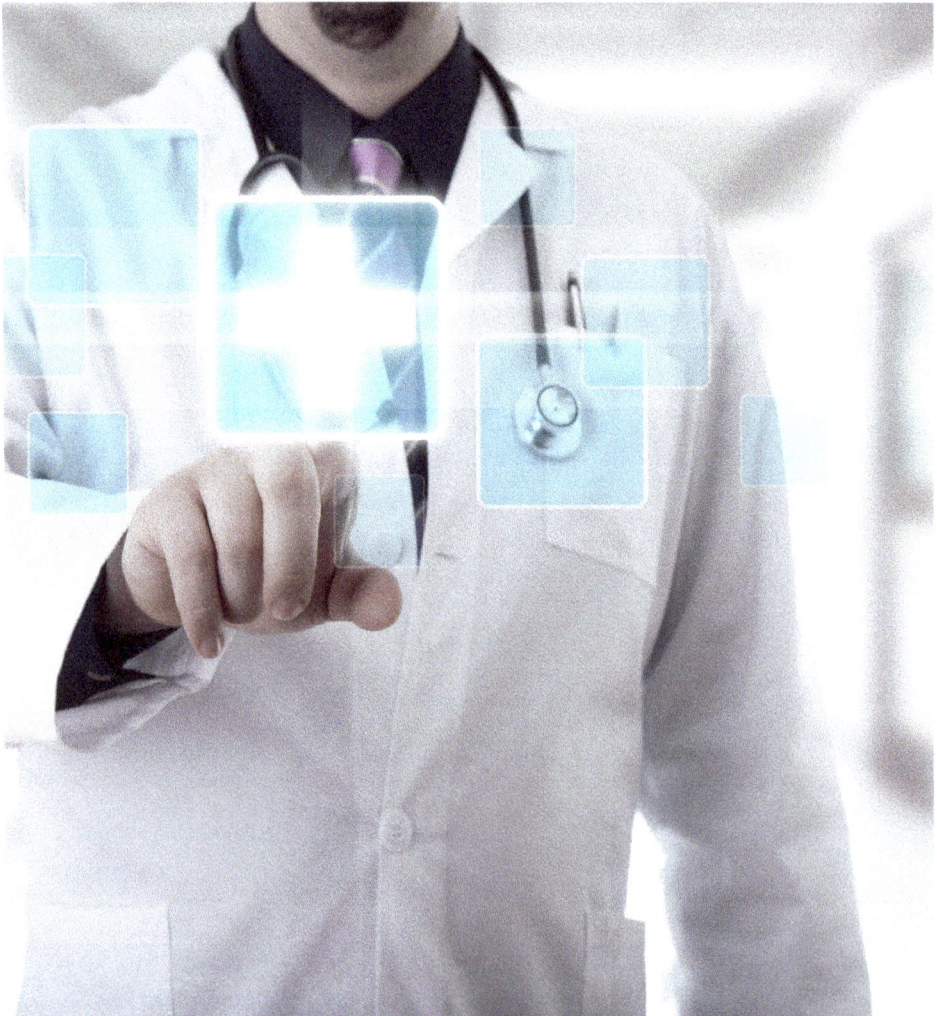

Purchasing

The intent of the Purchasing process is to ensure that purchased, sub-contracted, or otherwise received products and services conform to specified requirements. The medical device organization is expected to establish and maintain documented controls for planning and performing purchasing activities. The controls necessary depend on the effect of the product on the quality, safety, and effectiveness of the finished device. Effective purchasing processes incorporate purchasing requirements and specifications, the selection of acceptable suppliers based on the capability of the suppliers to provide acceptable product, the performance of necessary acceptance activities, and maintenance of the required quality records.

The management representative is responsible for ensuring that the requirements of the quality management system have been effectively defined, documented, implemented, and maintained. Prior to the audit of a process, it may be helpful to interview the management representative to obtain an overview of the process and a feel for management's knowledge and understanding of the process.

Clause and Regulation
ISO: ISO: ISO 13485:2016: 4.1.2, 4.1.3, 4.1.5, 7.1, 7.4.1, 7.4.2, 7.4.3

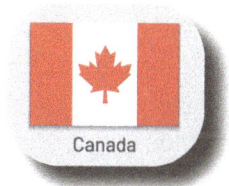

Canada

Planning

In planning product realization, the medical device organization must determine as appropriate the quality objectives and requirements for the purchased products, the processes, documents, and resources specific to the purchased products, the criteria for purchased product acceptance, and the required verification, monitoring, inspection, and test activities specific to the purchased products. Planning of product realization often begins in the design and development of the product, including the translation of the design into production specifications. The translation of the design into production specifications includes the establishment of specified requirements for purchased product.

Quality objectives

Quality objectives are typically expressed as a measurable target or goal. The planning of product realization should include consideration of how the purchased product, the criteria for purchased product acceptance, and the required verification, monitoring, inspection, and test activities specific to the purchased product will achieve the quality objectives.

- Some examples of QOB include:
- Number of complaints -v- number of parts shipped
- On-time delivery %
- Supplier parts rejected
- Comparison of internal audit findings -v- external audit findings
- Achieving a certain accuracy if you're developing product - based software
- Annual Post-market surveillance
- Auditing our system for regulatory compliance

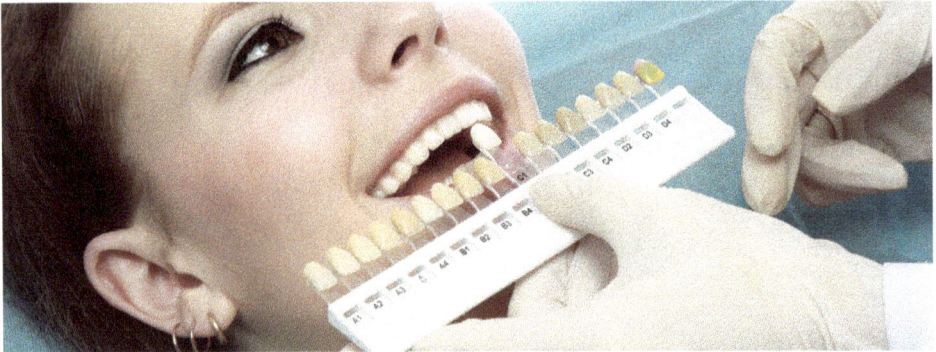

Some managers believe that the reward for hard work should be a paycheck. That's sort of like telling your children that they get to eat for doing something you're proud of. Employees are not children, but you are responsible for developing them into more valuable employees so that they can be promoted. If there is no incentive, your team will not be engaged. Therefore, pick a reward that is proportional to the bottom-line impact. Five percent of the bottom-line impact is what I like to target, but you would be amazed at how effective a few small rewards at each milestone can be. If you have trouble getting management approval for rewards, remind your boss of the bottom-line impact and link the rewards closely to the impact.

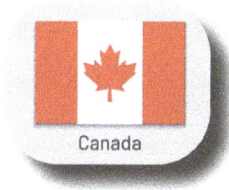

Canada

MDSAP
Audit Checklist

	REQUIREMENTS
	4 Quality management system
	4.1 General requirements
	Has the organization:
	a) identified the processes needed for the quality management system and their application throughout the organization (see 1.2)?
	b) determined the sequence and interaction of these processes?
	c) determined criteria and methods needed to ensure that both the operation and control of these processes are effective?
	d) ensured the availability of resources and information necessary to support the operation and monitoring of their processes?
	e) monitored, measured, and analyzed these processes
	f) implemented actions necessary to achieve planned results and maintain the effectiveness of these processes?
	Does the organization manage these processes in accordance with the requirements of this International Standard?
	Where an organization chooses to outsource any process that affects product conformity with requirements, does the organization ensure control over such processes?
	Is the control of such outsourced processes identified within the quality management system? (see 8.5.1)
Canada	Verify that the roles and responsibilities of any regulatory correspondents, importers, distributors, or providers of a service are clearly documented in the organization's quality management system and are qualified as suppliers and controlled.
	4.2.1 General

Doc. Reference	Adequate?	Stage I (clauses marked *)	Stage II
	Y/N	Initial›s	Initial›s

	REQUIREMENTS
	Does the quality management system documentation include:
	a) documented statements of a quality policy and quality objectives?
	b) a quality manual?
	c) documented procedures required by this international standard?
	d) documents needed by the organization to ensure the effective planning, operation and control of its processes?
	e) records required by this International Standard (see 4.2.4)?
	f) any other documentation specified by national or regional regulations?
	Has the organization established and maintained a file for each type or model of medical device either containing or identifying documents defining product specifications and quality system requirements (see 4.2.3)?
	Do these documents define the complete manufacturing process and, if applicable, installation and servicing?
Canada	With respect to Class II devices that are not subject to Design and Development controls, verify that the manufacturer has objective evidence to establish that Class II devices meet the safety and effectiveness requirements of section 10 to 20 [CMDR 10 ,9 to 20].

Doc. Reference	Adequate?	Stage I (clauses marked *)	Stage II

	REQUIREMENTS	
Canada	Verify that the manufacturer maintains distribution records that contain sufficient information to permit complete and rapid withdrawal of the medical device from the market [CMDR 53-52].	
	Verify that distribution records of a device are retained by the manufacturer in a manner that will allow for timely retrieval, for the longer of (a) the projected useful life of the device; and (b) two years after the date the device was shipped [CMDR 56-55].	
EU	Does the file contain or refer to the location of objective evidence establishing the safety and effectiveness of the device as required by Annex 1 of the MDD? (MDD Annex I)	
4.2.2 Quality manual		
	Has the organization established and maintained a quality manual that includes:	
	a) the scope of the quality management system, including details of and justification for any exclusion and/or non-application (see 1.2)?	
	b) the documented procedures established for the quality management system, or reference to them?	
	c) a description of the interaction between the processes of the quality management system?	
	Does the quality manual outline the structure of the documentation used in the quality management system?	
Canada	Verify that the manufacturer has defined, documented, and implemented processes to ensure that devices are licensed prior to sale [CMDR Sections 43 ,34 ,32 ,26	
	Verify that the manufacturer has defined, documented and implemented processes to ensure that any new or modified quality management system certificate issued to the manufacturer for regulatory purposes is submitted to the Minister within 30 days after it is issued [CMDR Section 43.1].	

Doc. Reference	Adequate?	Stage I (clauses marked *)	Stage II

	REQUIREMENTS
EU	Are the applicable sections of the Medical Device Directive (MDD) included in the specified requirements throughout the documented quality system? Interpretation: A statement only indicating compliance/conformity with the relevant international or EU regulatory requirements is not acceptable.
4.2.3 Control of documents	
	Are documents required by the quality management system controlled?
	Is a documented procedure established to define the controls needed:
	a) To review and approve documents for adequacy prior to issue?
	b) To review and update as necessary and re-approve documents?
	c) To ensure that changes and the current revision status of documents are identified?
	d) To ensure that relevant versions of applicable documents are available at points of use?
	e) To ensure the documents remain legible and readily identifiable?
	f) To ensure that documents of external origin are identified and their distribution controlled?
	g) To prevent the unintended use of obsolete documents and to apply suitable identification to them if they are retained for any purpose?
	Does the organization ensure that changes to documents are reviewed and approved either by the original approving function or another designated function which has access to pertinent background information upon which to base its decisions?

Doc. Reference	Adequate?	Stage I (clauses marked *)	Stage II

	REQUIREMENTS
	Does the organization define the period for which at least one copy of obsolete controlled documents shall be retained?
	Does this period ensure that documents to which medical devices have been manufactured and tested are available for at least the lifetime of the medical device as defined by the organization, but not less than the retention period of any resulting record (see 4.2.4), or as specified by relevant regulatory requirements?
4.2.4 Control of quality records	
	Are records established and maintained to provide evidence of conformity to requirements and of the effective operation of the quality management system?
	Do records remain legible, readily identifiable and retrievable?
	Has a documented procedure been established to define the controls needed for the identification, storage, protection, retrieval, retention time and disposition of records?
	Does the organization retain the records for a period of time at least equivalent to the lifetime of the medical device as defined by the organization, but not less than two years from the date of product release by the organization or as specified by relevant regulatory requirements?
EU	Has the manufacturer retained for a period ending at least five years after the last product has been manufactured, the records listed in Annex II, 6.1 or Annex V, 5.1 or Annex VI, 5.1 (whichever applies)
5 Management responsibility	
5.1 Management commitment	

Doc. Reference	Adequate?	Stage I (clauses marked *)	Stage II

	REQUIREMENTS	
	Has top management provided evidence of its commitment to the development and implementation of the quality management system and maintaining its effectiveness by:	
	a) Communicating to the organization the importance of meeting customer as well as statutory and regulatory requirements?	
	b) Establishing the quality policy?	
	c) Ensuring that quality objectives are established?	
	d) Conducting management reviews?	
	e) Ensuring the availability of resources?	
5.2 Customer focus		
	Does top management ensure that customer requirements are determined and met (see 7.2.1 and 8.2.1)?	
5.3 Quality policy		
	Does top management ensure that the quality policy	
	a) Is appropriate to the purpose of the organization?	
	b) Includes a commitment to comply with requirements and to maintain the effectiveness of the quality management system?	
	c) Provides a framework for establishing and reviewing quality objectives?	
	d) Is communicated and understood within the organization?	
	e) Is reviewed for continuing suitability?	
5.4 Planning		
5.4.1 Quality objectives		
	Does top management ensure that quality objectives, including those needed to meet requirements for product (see 7.1a), are established at relevant functions and levels within the organization?	
	Are quality objectives measurable?	

Doc. Reference	Adequate?	Stage I (clauses marked *)	Stage II

	REQUIREMENTS
	Are quality objectives consistent with the quality policy?
5.4.2 Quality management system planning	
	Has top management ensured that:
	a) The planning of the quality management system is carried out in order to meet the requirements given in 4.1, as well as the quality objectives?
	b) The integrity of the quality management system is maintained when changes to the quality management system are planned and implemented?
5.5 Responsibility, authority and communication	
5.5.1 Responsibility and authority	
	Has top management ensured that responsibilities and authorities were defined, documented and communicated within the organization?
	Has top management established the interrelation of all personnel who manage, perform and verify work affecting quality, and ensured the independence and authority necessary to perform these tasks?
5.5.2 Management representative	
	Has top management appointed a member of management who, irrespective of other responsibilities, has responsibility and authority that includes:
	a) Ensuring that processes needed for the quality management system are established, implemented, and maintained?
	b) Reporting to top management on the performance of the quality management system and any need for improvement (see 8.5)?
	c) Ensuring the promotion of awareness of regulatory and customer requirements throughout the organization?
5.5.3 Internal communication	

Doc. Reference	Adequate?	Stage I (clauses marked *)	Stage II

	REQUIREMENTS
	Has top management ensured that appropriate communication processes have been established within the organization and that communication takes place regarding the effectiveness of the quality management system?
5.6 Management review	
5.6.1 General	
	Does top management review the organization's quality management system, at planned intervals, to ensure its continuing suitability, adequacy and effectiveness?
	Does this review include assessing opportunities for improvement and the need for changes to the quality management system, including the quality policy and quality objectives?
	Are records from management reviews maintained (see 4.2.4)?
5.6.2 Review input	
	Does the input to management review include information on:
	a) Results of audits?
	b) Customer feedback?
	c) Process performance and product conformity?
	d) Status of preventive and corrective actions?
	e) Follow-up actions from previous management reviews?
	f) Changes that could affect the quality management system?
	g) Recommendations for improvement?
	h) New or revised regulatory requirements?
5.6.3 Review output	

Doc. Reference	Adequate?	Stage I (clauses marked *)	Stage II

	REQUIREMENTS	
	Does output from the management review include any decisions and actions related to:	
	a) Improvements needed to maintain the effectiveness of the quality management system and its processes?	
	b) Improvement of product related to customer requirements?	
	c) Resource needs?	
6 Resource management		
6.1 Provision of resources		
	Does the organization determine and provide the resources needed:	
	a) To implement the quality management system and to maintain its effectiveness?	
	b) To meet regulatory and customer requirements?	
6.2 Human resources		
6.2.1 General		
	Are personnel performing work affecting product quality competent on the basis of appropriate education, training, skills and experience?	
6.2.2 Competence, awareness and training		
	Does the organization:	
	a) determine the necessary competence for personnel performing work affecting product quality?	
	b) Provide training or take other actions to satisfy these needs?	
	c) Evaluate the effectiveness of actions taken?	
	d) Ensure that its personnel are aware of the relevance and importance of their activities and how they contribute to the achievement of the quality objectives?	
	e) Maintain appropriate records of education, training, skills and experience (see 4.2.4)?	

Doc. Reference	Adequate?	Stage I (clauses marked *)	Stage II

	REQUIREMENTS
US	Verify that resources include the assignment of trained personnel to meet the requirements of 21 CFR Part 820, including management, performance of work, assessment activities, and internal quality audits [21 CFR 820.20(b)(2)].
6.3 Infrastructure	
	Does the organization determine, provide and maintain the infrastructure needed to achieve conformity to product requirements?
	Infrastructure includes, as applicable:
	a) Buildings, workspace and associated utilities
	b) Process equipment, both hardware and software
	c) Supporting services such as transport or communication
	Does the organization establish documented requirements for maintenance activities, including their frequency, when such activities or lack thereof can affect product quality?
	Are records of such maintenance maintained (see 4.2.4)?
	Has the organization determined and does it manage the work environment needed to achieve conformity to product requirements?
	a) Has the organization established documented requirements for health, cleanliness and clothing of personnel if contact between such personnel and the product or work environment could adversely affect the quality of the product (see 7.5.1.2.1)?
	b) If work environment conditions can have an adverse effect on product quality, has organization established documented requirements for the work environment conditions and documented procedures or work instructions to monitor and control these work environment conditions (see 7.5.1.2.1)?

Doc. Reference	Adequate?	Stage I (clauses marked *)	Stage II

	REQUIREMENTS
	c) Does the organization ensure that all personnel who are required to work temporarily under special environmental conditions within the work environment are appropriately trained or supervised by a trained person [see 6.2.2 b)]?
	d) If appropriate, are special arrangements established and documented for the control of contaminated or potentially contaminated product in order to prevent contamination of other product, the work environment or personnel (see 7.5.3.1)?
7 Product realization	
7.1 Planning of product realization	
	Has the organization planned and developed the processes needed for product realization?
	Is the planning of product realization consistent with the requirements of the other processes of the quality management system (see 4.1)?
	In planning product realization, has the organization determined the following, as appropriate:
	a) Quality objectives and requirements for products?
	b) The need to establish processes, documents, and provide resources specific to the product?
	c) Required verification, validation, monitoring, inspection and test activities specific to the product and the criteria for product acceptance?
	d) Records needed to provide evidence that the realization processes and resulting product meet requirements (see 4.2.4)?
	Is the output of this planning in a form suitable for the organization's method of operations?

Doc. Reference	Adequate?	Stage I (clauses marked *)	Stage II

	REQUIREMENTS
	Does the organization establish documented requirements for risk management throughout product realization and are records arising from risk management maintained (see 4.2.4)?
Canada	Verify that the manufacturer has a process or procedure for identifying a "significant change" to a class III or IV device. Verify that information about "significant changes" is submitted in a medical device license amendment application [CMDR 34 ,1].
EU	Does the supplier evaluate the need for risk analysis throughout the design process and maintain records of any risk analysis performed? (MDD Annex 1)

7.2.1 Determination of requirements related to the product	
	Has the organization determined:
	a) Requirements specified by the customer, including the requirements for delivery and post-delivery activities?
	b) Requirements not stated by the customer but necessary for specified or intended use, where known?
	c) Statutory and regulatory requirements related to the product?
	d) Any additional requirements determined by the organization?

Doc. Reference	Adequate?	Stage I (clauses marked *)	Stage II

	REQUIREMENTS
Canada	Verify that the manufacturer has met the device licensing requirements prior to mport or sell a Class II, III or IV medical device in Canada [CMDR 32]. Manufacturer means a person who sells a medical device under their own name, or under a trade-mark, design, trade name or other name or mark owned or controlled by the person, and who is responsible for designing, manufacturing, assembling, processing, labeling, packaging, refurbishing or modifying the device, or for assigning to it a purpose, whether those tasks are performed by that person or on their behalf [CMDR 1]. No person shall import or sell a Class II, III or IV medical device unless the manufacturer of the device holds a license in respect of that device or, if the medical device has been subjected to a change described in section 34, an amended medical device license [CMDR 26]. An application for a medical device license shall be submitted to the Minister by the manufacturer of the medical device in a format established by the Minister [CMDR 32]. An application for a medical device license shall include a copy of a quality management system certificate certifying that the quality management system under which the medical device is manufactured (class II) or designed and manufacturer (class III or IV) satisfies National Standard of Canada CAN/CSA-ISO 13485:2003. [CMDR 2)32)(f); 3)32)(j); 4)32)(p)].

Doc. Reference	Adequate?	Stage I (clauses marked *)	Stage II

	REQUIREMENTS
EU	Vefiy that manufacturing maintains files containing or refer to the location of objective evidence establishing the safety and effectiveness of the device as required by Annex 1 of the MDD. Verify that the manufacturer followed a defined and effective process to establish and maintain a file containing documents defining product specifications and quality system requirements for each newa and existing type/modes of medical devices. Since the last audit, has the manufacturer introduced new products in the EU? Has the manufacturer followed a defined and effective process to obtain an approval from the Notified Body to CE mark a product prior to selling it in the EU? (does not apply to class I devices)
7.2.2 Review of requirements related to the product	
	Does the organization review the requirements related to the product?
	Is this review conducted prior to the organization's commitment to supply a product to the customer (e.g. submission of tenders, acceptance of contracts or orders, acceptance of changes to contracts or orders)?
	Does the organization ensure that:
	a) Product requirements are defined and documented?
	b) Contract or order requirements differing from those previously expressed are resolved?
	c) The organization has the ability to meet the defined requirements?
	Are records of the results of the review and actions arising from the review maintained (see 4.2.4)?

Doc. Reference	Adequate?	Stage I (clauses marked *)	Stage II

	REQUIREMENTS	
	Where the customer provides no documented statement of requirement, are the customer requirements confirmed by the organization before acceptance?	
	Where product requirements are changed, does the organization ensure that relevant documents are amended and that relevant personnel are made aware of the changed requirements?	
7.2.3 Customer communication		
	Has the organization determined and implemented effective arrangements for communicating with customers in relation to:	
	a) Product information?	
	b) Enquiries, contracts or order handling, including amendments?	
	c) Customer feedback, including customer complaints? (see 8.2.1)	
	d) Advisory notices? (see 8.5.1)	
7.3 Design and development		
7.3.1 Design and/or development planning		
	Has the organization established documented procedures for design and development?	
	Does the organization plan and control the design and development of product?	
	During the design and development planning, does the organization determine:	
	a) The design and development stages?	
	b) The review, verification, validation and design transfer activities (see Note) that are appropriate at each design and development stage?	
	c) The responsibilities and authorities for design and development?	

Doc. Reference	Adequate?	Stage I (clauses marked *)	Stage II

	REQUIREMENTS
	Does the organization manage the interfaces between different groups involved in design and development to ensure effective communication and clear assignment of responsibility?
	Is planning output documented, and updated as appropriate, as the design and development progresses? (See 4.2.3)
Canada	Verify that manufacturers of Class IV devices maintain a quality plan that sets out the specific quality practices, resources, and sequence of activities relevant to the device [CMDR 32].
7.3.2 Design and development inputs	
	Have inputs relating to product requirements been determined and records maintained (see 4.2.4)?
	Do these inputs include:
	a) Functional, performance and safety requirements, according to the intended use?
	b) Applicable statutory and regulatory requirements?
	c) Where applicable, information derived from previous similar designs?
	d) Other requirements essential for design and development?
	e) Output(s) of risk management (see 7.1)?
	Are these inputs reviewed for adequacy and approved?
	Are requirements complete, unambiguous and not in conflict with each other?
7.3.3 Design and development outputs	
	Are the outputs of design and development provided in a form that enables verification against the design and development input, and is it approved prior to release?

Doc. Reference	Adequate?	Stage I (clauses marked *)	Stage II

	REQUIREMENTS
	Do design and development outputs:
	a) meet the input requirements for design and development?
	b) Provide appropriate information for purchasing, production and for service provision?
	c) Contain or reference product acceptance criteria?
	d) Specify the characteristics of the product that are essential for its safe and proper use?
	Are records of the design and development outputs maintained (see 4.2.4)?
7.3.4 Design and development review	
	At suitable stages, are systematic reviews of design and development performed in accordance with planned arrangements (see 7.3.1):
	a) To evaluate the ability of the results of design and development to meet requirements?
	b) To identify any problems and propose necessary actions?
	Do participants in such reviews include representatives of functions concerned with the design and development stage(s) being reviewed, as well as other specialist personnel (see 5.5.1 and 6.2.1)?
	Are records of the results of the reviews and any necessary actions maintained (see 4.2.4)?
EU	Does the supplier evaluate the need for risk analysis throughout the design process and maintain records of any risk analysis performed? (MDD Annex 1)
7.3.5 Design and development verification	
	Is verification performed in accordance with planned arrangements (see 7.3.1) to ensure that the design and development outputs have met the design and development input requirements?
	Are records of the results of the verification and any necessary actions maintained?

Doc. Reference	Adequate?	Stage I (clauses marked *)	Stage II

	REQUIREMENTS
7.3.6 Design and development validation	
	Is design and development validation performed in accordance with planned arrangements (see 7.3.1) to ensure that the resulting product is capable of meeting the requirements for the specified application or intended use?
	Is validation completed prior to the delivery or implementation of the product (see Note 1)?
	Are records of the results of validation and any necessary actions maintained (see 4.2.4)?
	As part of design and development validation, does the organization perform clinical evaluations and/or evaluation of performance of the medical device, as required by national or regional regulations (see Note 2)?
7.3.7 Control of design and development changes	
	Are design and development changes identified and records maintained?
	Are changes reviewed, verified, and validated, as appropriate, and approved before implementation?
	Does the review of design and development changes include evaluation of the effect of the changes on constituent parts and product already delivered?
	Are records of the results of the review of changes and any necessary actions maintained?
Canada	Verify that the manufacturer has a process or procedure for identifying a "significant change" to a Class III or IV medical device. Verify that information about "significant changes" is submitted in a medical device licenseamendment application [CMDR 34 ,1].
EU	Do documented procedures identify the need to report essential changes to the Notified Body, (MDD Annex II, V, VI, 3.4)

Doc. Reference	Adequate?	Stage I (clauses marked *)	Stage II

	REQUIREMENTS

7.4 Purchasing	
7.4.1 Purchasing process	
	Has the organization established documented procedures to ensure that purchased product conforms to specified purchase requirements?
	Is the type and extent of control applied to the supplier and the purchased product dependent upon the effect of the purchased product on subsequent product realization or the final product?
	Does the organization evaluate and select suppliers based on their ability to supply product in accordance with the organization's requirements?
	Have criteria for selection, evaluation and re-evaluation been established?
	Are records of the results of evaluation and any necessary actions arising from the evaluation maintained (see 4.2.4)?
Canada	Verify that any regulatory correspondent used by the manufacturer is treated as a supplier and is adequately qualified.
7.4.2 Purchasing information	
	Does purchasing information describe the product to be purchased, including where appropriate:
	a) Requirements for approval of product, procedures, processes and equipment?
	b) Requirements for qualification of personnel?
	c) Quality management system requirements?
	Does the organization ensure the adequacy of specified purchase requirements prior to their communication to the supplier?
	To the extent required for traceability given in 7.5.3.2, does the organization maintain relevant purchasing information, i.e. documents (see 4.2.3) and records (see 4.2.4)?

Doc. Reference	Adequate?	Stage I (clauses marked *)	Stage II

	REQUIREMENTS
7.4.3 Verification of purchased product	
	Has the organization established and implemented the inspection or other activities necessary for ensuring that purchased product meets specified purchase requirements?
	Where the organization or its customer intends to perform verification at the supplier's premises, does the organization state the intended verification arrangements and method of product release in the purchasing information?
	Are records of the verification maintained (see 4.2.4)?
7.5 Production and service provision	
7.5.1 Control of production and service provision	
7.5.1.1 General Requirements	
	Does the organization plan and carry out production and service provision under controlled conditions?
	Do the controlled conditions include, as applicable:
	a) The availability of information that describes the characteristics of the product?
	b) The availability of documented procedures, documented requirements, work instructions, reference materials and reference measurement procedures as necessary?
	c) The use of suitable equipment?
	d) The availability and use of monitoring and measuring devices?
	e) The implementation of monitoring and measurement?
	f) The implementation of release, delivery and post-delivery activities?
	g) The implementation of defined operations for labeling and packaging?

Doc. Reference	Adequate?	Stage I (clauses marked *)	Stage II

	REQUIREMENTS	
	Does the organization establish and maintain a record (see 4.2.4) for each batch of medical devices that provides traceability to the extent specified in 7.5.3 and identifies the amount manufactured and amount approved for distribution?	
	Is the batch record verified and approved?	
7.5.1.2 Control of production and service provision — Specific requirements		
7.5.1.2.1 Cleanliness of product and contamination control		
	Does the organization establish documented requirements for cleanliness of product if:	
	a) Product is cleaned by the organization prior to sterilization and/or its use, or	
	b) Product is supplied non-sterile to be subjected to a cleaning process prior to sterilization and/or its use, or	
	c) Product is supplied to be used non-sterile and its cleanliness is of significance in use, or	
	d) Process agents are to be removed from product during manufacture?	
	If product is cleaned in accordance with a) or b) above, the requirements contained in 6.4 a) and 6.4 b) do not apply prior to the cleaning process.	
7.5.1.2.2 Installation activities		
	If appropriate, does the organization establish documented requirements which contain acceptance criteria for installing and verifying the installation of the medical device?	
	If the agreed customer requirements allow installation to be performed other than by the organization or its authorized agent, does the organization provide documented requirements for installation and verification?	
	Are records of installation and verification performed by the organization or its authorized agent maintained (see 4.2.4)?	

Doc. Reference	Adequate?	Stage I (clauses marked *)	Stage II

	REQUIREMENTS

7.5.1.2.3 Servicing activities	
	If servicing is a specified requirement, does the organization establish documented procedures, work instructions and reference materials and reference measurement procedures, as necessary, for performing servicing activities and verifying that they meet the specified requirements?
	Are records of servicing activities carried out by the organization maintained (see 4.2.4)?

7.5.1.3 Particular requirements for sterile medical devices	
	Does the organization maintain records of the process parameters for the sterilization process which was used for each sterilization batch (see 4.2.4)?
	Are sterilization records traceable to each production batch of medical devices (see 7.5.1.1)?

7.5.2 Validation of processes for production and service provision	

7.5.2.1 General requirements	
	Does the organization validate any processes for production and service provision where the resulting output cannot be verified by subsequent monitoring or measurement? (this includes any processes where deficiencies become apparent only after the product is in use or the service has been delivered)
	Does validation demonstrate the ability of the processes to achieve planned results?
	Has the organization established arrangements for these processes including, as applicable:
	a) Defined criteria for review and approval of the processes?
	b) Approval of equipment and qualification of personnel?
	c) Use of specific methods and procedures?
	d) Requirements for records (see 4.2.4)?
	e) Re-validation?

Doc. Reference	Adequate?	Stage I (clauses marked *)	Stage II

	REQUIREMENTS
	Has the organization established documented procedures for the validation of the application of computer software (and changes to such software and/or its application) for production and service provision that affect the ability of the product to conform to specified requirements?
	Are such software applications validated prior to initial use?
	Are records of validation maintained (see 4.2.4)?
7.5.2.2 Particular requirements for sterile medical devices	
	Has the organization established documented procedures for the validation of sterilization processes?
	Are sterilization processes validated prior to initial use?
	Are records of validation of each sterilization process maintained (see 4.2.4)?
Canada	Verify that sterilization methods for devices sold in a sterile state are validated [CMDR 17].
7.5.3 Identification and traceability	
7.5.3.1 Identification	
	Does the organization identify the product by suitable means throughout product realization and does the organization establish documented procedures for such product identification?
	Has the organization established documented procedures to ensure that medical devices returned to the organization are identified and distinguished from conforming product [see 6.4 d)]?
7.5.3.2 Traceability	
7.5.3.2.1 General	
	Has the organization established documented procedures for traceability?
	Do such procedures define the extent of product traceability and the records required (see 8.3 ,4.2.4 and 8.5)?

Doc. Reference	Adequate?	Stage I (clauses marked *)	Stage II

	REQUIREMENTS	
	Does the organization control and record the unique identification of the product, where traceability is a requirement (see 4.2.4)?	
Canada	Verify that the manufacturer maintains objective evidence that devices meet the safety and effectiveness requirements of the CMDR [CMDR 2)9)]. Verify that devices sold in Canada have labeling that conforms to Canadian English and French language requirements and contains the manufacturer's name and address, device identifier, control number (for Class III and IV devices), contents of packaging, sterility, expiry, intended use, directions for use and any special storage conditions [CMDR 23-21].	
EU	Does the manufacturer have procedures identifying the requirements of labeling and instructions for use as defined in MDD, Annex 1 point 13, and is regulations for CE marking included in these procedures. (MDD 3, Article 17 and Annex 12).	
	Are language requirements defined in procedures for the information identified in MDD, Annex 1point 13 for the applicable markets.	
7.5.3.2.2 Particular requirements for active implantable medical devices and		
	In defining the records required for traceability, does the organization include records of all components, materials and work environment conditions, if these could cause the medical device not to satisfy its specified requirements?	
	Does the organization require that its agents or distributors maintain records of the distribution of medical devices to allow traceability and that such records be available for inspection?	

Doc. Reference	Adequate?	Stage I (clauses marked *)	Stage II

e medical devices

	REQUIREMENTS
	Are records of the name and address of the shipping package consignee maintained (see 4.2.4)?
Canada	Verify that the manufacturer has identified Schedule 2 implants and provides implant registration cards with devices or employs another suitable system approved by Health Canada [CMDR 68-66]. Verify that the manufacturer of devices that are listed on Schedule 2 of the Medical Devices Regulations maintains distribution records of these devices as well as any information received on implant registration cards related to these Schedule 2 devices [CMDR 54].
7.5.3.3 Status identification	
	Does the organization identify the product status with respect to monitoring and measurement requirements?
	Is the identification of product status maintained throughout production, storage, installation and servicing of the product to ensure that only product that has passed the required inspections and tests (or released under an authorized concession) is dispatched, used or installed?
7.5.4 Customer property	
	Does the organization exercise care with customer property while it is under the organization's control or being used by the organization?
	Does the organization identify, verify, protect and safeguard customer property provided for use or incorporation into the product?
	If any customer property is lost, damaged, or otherwise found to be unsuitable for use, is this reported to the customer and are records maintained (see 4.2.4)?
7.5.5 Preservation of product	

Doc. Reference	Adequate?	Stage I (clauses marked *)	Stage II

	REQUIREMENTS
	Has the organization established documented procedures or documented work instructions for preserving the conformity of product during internal processing and delivery to the intended destination?
	Does this preservation include identification, handling, packaging, storage and protection, and also apply to the constituent parts of a product?
	Has the organization established documented procedures or documented work instructions for the control of product with a limited shelf-life or requiring special storage conditions?
	Are such special storage conditions controlled and recorded (see 4.2.4)?
7.6 Control of monitoring and measuring devices	
	Does the organization determine monitoring and measuring to be undertaken and the monitoring and measuring devices needed to provide evidence of conformity of product to determined requirements (guide reference 7.2.1)?
	Has the organization established documented procedures to ensure that monitoring and measurement can be carried out and are carried out in a manner that is consistent with the monitoring and measurement requirements?

Doc. Reference	Adequate?	Stage I (clauses marked *)	Stage II

	REQUIREMENTS
	Where necessary to ensure valid results, is measuring equipment:
	a) Calibrated or verified at specified intervals, or prior to use, against measurement standards traceable to international or national measurement standards; where no such standards exist, is the basis used for calibration or verification recorded?
	b) Adjusted or re-adjusted as necessary?
	c) Identified to enable the calibration status to be determined?
	d) Safeguarded from adjustments that would invalidate the measurement result?
	e) Protected from damage and deterioration during handling, maintenance and storage?
	Does the organization assess and record the validity of the previous measuring results when the equipment is found not to conform to requirements?
	Does the organization take appropriate action on the equipment and any product affected?
	Are records of the results of calibration and verification maintained (see 4.2.4)?
	When used in the monitoring and measurement of specified requirements, is the ability of computer software to satisfy the intended application confirmed prior to initial use and reconfirmed as necessary ?
8 Measurement, analysis and improvement	
8.1 General	

Doc. Reference	Adequate?	Stage I (clauses marked *)	Stage II

	REQUIREMENTS
	Does the organization plan and implement the monitoring, measurement, analysis and improvement processes needed:
	a) To demonstrate conformity of the product?
	b) To ensure conformity of the quality management system?
	c) To maintain the effectiveness of the quality management system?
	Does this include determination of applicable methods, including statistical techniques, and the extent of their use?
8.2 Monitoring and measurement	
8.2.1 Feedback	
	As one of the measurements of the performance of the quality management system, does the organization monitor information relating to whether the organization has met customer requirements?
	Have the methods for obtaining and using this information been determined?
	Has the organization established a documented procedure for a feedback system [see 7.2.3 c)] to provide early warning of quality problems and for input into the corrective and preventive action processes (see 8.5.2 and 8.5.3)?
	If national or regional regulations require the organization to gain experience from the post-production phase, does the review of this experience form part of the feedback system (see 8.5.1)?

Doc. Reference	Adequate?	Stage I (clauses marked *)	Stage II

	REQUIREMENTS
Canada	Verify that the manufacturer maintains records of reported problems related to the performance characteristics or safety of a device, including any consumer complaints received by the manufacturer after the device was first sold in Canada, and all actions taken by the manufacturer in response to the problems referred to in t hecomplaints [CMDR Section 57]. Verify that the manufacturer has established and implemented documented procedures that will enable it to carry out an effective and timely investigation of the problems reports through the customer complaints, andto carry out an effective and timely recall of the device [CMDR Section 58].
8.2.2 Internal audit	
	Does the organization conduct internal audits at planned intervals to determine whether the quality management system
	a) Conforms to the planned arrangements (see 7.1), to the requirements of this International Standard and to the quality management system requirements established by the organization?
	b) Is effectively implemented and maintained?
	Is an audit programme planned, taking into consideration the status and importance of the processes and areas to be audited, as well as the results of previous audits?
	Are the audit criteria, scope, frequency and methods defined?
	Does selection of auditors and conduct of audits ensure objectivity and impartiality of the audit process (e.g. auditors shall not audit their own work)?
	Are the responsibilities and requirements for planning and conducting audits, and for reporting results and maintaining records (see 4.2.4) defined in a documented procedure?

Doc. Reference	Adequate?	Stage I (clauses marked *)	Stage II

	REQUIREMENTS
	Does management responsible for the area being audited ensure that actions are taken without undue delay to eliminate detected nonconformities and their causes?
	Do follow-up activities include the verification of the actions taken and the reporting of verification results? (see 8.5.2)
8.2.3 Measurement and monitoring of processes	
	Does the organization apply suitable methods for monitoring and, where applicable, measurement of the quality management system processes?
	Do these methods demonstrate the ability of the processes to achieve planned results?
	When planned results are not achieved, is correction and corrective action taken, as appropriate, to ensure conformity of the product?
8.2.4 Monitoring and measurement of product	
8.2.4.1 General requirements	
	Does the organization monitor and measure the characteristics of the product to verify that product requirements have been met?
	Is this carried out at appropriate stages of the product realization process in accordance with the planned arrangements (see 7.1) and documented procedures (see 7.5.1.1)?
	Is evidence of conformity with the acceptance criteria maintained?
	Do records indicate the person(s) authorizing release of the product (see 4.2.4)?
	Does the organization ensure that product release and service delivery do not proceed until the planned arrangements (see 7.1) have been satisfactorily completed?
8.2.4.2 Particular requirement for active implantable medical devices and im

Doc. Reference	Adequate?	Stage I (clauses marked *)	Stage II
medical devices			

	REQUIREMENTS
	Does the organization record (see 4.2.4) the identity of personnel performing any inspection or testing?
8.3 Control of nonconforming product	
	Does the organization ensure that product which does not conform to product requirements is identified and controlled to prevent its unintended use or delivery?
	Are the controls and related responsibilities and authorities for dealing with nonconforming product defined in a documented procedure?
	Does the organization deal with nonconforming product by one or more of the following ways?
	a) By taking action to eliminate the detected nonconformity
	b) By authorizing its use, release or acceptance under concession
	c) By taking action to preclude its original intended use or application
	Does the organization ensure that nonconforming product is accepted by concession only if regulatory requirements are met?
	Are records of the identity of the person(s) authorizing the concession maintained (see 4.2.4)?
	Are records of the nature of nonconformities and any subsequent actions taken, including concessions obtained maintained (see 4.2.4)?
	When nonconforming product is corrected, is it subject to re-verification to demonstrate conformity to the requirements?
	When nonconforming product is detected after delivery or use has started, does the organization take action appropriate to the effects, or potential effects, of the nonconformity?

Doc. Reference	Adequate?	Stage I (clauses marked *)	Stage II

	REQUIREMENTS
	If product needs to be reworked (one or more times), does the organization document the rework process in a work instruction that has undergone the same authorization and approval procedure as the original work instruction?
	Prior to authorization and approval of the work instruction, is a determination of any adverse effect of the rework upon product made and documented (see 4.2.3 and 7.5.1)?
8.4 Analysis of data	
	Does the organization establish documented procedures to determine, collect and analyse appropriate data to demonstrate the suitability and effectiveness of the quality management system and to evaluate if improvement of the effectiveness of the quality management system can be made?
	Does this include data generated as a result of monitoring and measurement and from other relevant sources?
	Does the analysis of data provide information relating to:
	a) Feedback (see 8.2.1)?
	b) Conformity to product requirements? (See 7.2.1)
	c) Characteristics and trends of processes and products including opportunities for preventive action?
	d) Suppliers?
	Are records of the results of the analysis of data maintained (see 4.2.4)?
8.5 Improvement	
8.5.1 General	
	Does the organization identify and implement any changes necessary to ensure and maintain the continued suitability and effectiveness of the quality management system through the use of the quality policy, quality objectives, audit results, analysis of data, corrective and preventive actions and management review?

Doc. Reference	Adequate?	Stage I (clauses marked *)	Stage II

	REQUIREMENTS	
	Does the organization establish documented procedures for the issue and implementation of advisory notices and are these procedures capable of being implemented at any time?	
Canada	Verify the manufacturer has established procedures for reporting of recalls compliant with: [CMDR 65.1 – 63 ,1 Guide to Recall of Medical Devices GUI0054-]	
EU	Are the procedures for Vigilance reporting in conformance with MDD Annex II, V, and VI (MEDDEV 1-2.12)	
	Are records of all customer complaint investigations maintained (see 4.2.4)?	
	If investigation determines that the activities outside the organization contributed to the customer complaint, is relevant information exchanged between the organizations involved (see 4.1)?	
	If any customer complaint is not followed by corrective and/ or preventive action, is the reason authorized (see 5.5.1) and recorded (see 4.2.4)?	
	If national or regional regulations require notification of adverse events that meet specific reporting criteria, does the organization establish documented procedures to such notification to regulatory authorities?	
Canada	Verify that the manufacturer has established and implemented procedures compliant with requirements of: [Medical Device Regulations SOR/282-98, Section 61.1-59: Guidance Document for Mandatory Problem Reporting for Medical Devices]	
EU	Are procedures for the reporting of recall to the relevant competent authority and the NB compliant? (MDD, Annex II, V, VI, 3.1)	
8.5.2 Corrective action		

Doc. Reference	Adequate?	Stage I (clauses marked *)	Stage II

	REQUIREMENTS
	Does the organization take action to eliminate the cause of nonconformities in order to prevent recurrence and are corrective actions appropriate to the effects of the nonconformities encountered?
	Has a documented procedure been established to define requirements for:
	a) Reviewing nonconformities (including customer complaints)?
	b) Determining the causes of nonconformities?
	c) Evaluating the need for action to ensure that nonconformities do no recur?
	d) Determining and implementing action needed, including, if appropriate, updating documentation (see 4.2)?
	e) Recording of the results of any investigation and of action taken (see 4.2.4)?
	f) Reviewing the corrective action taken and its effectiveness?
8.5.3 Preventive action	
	Does the organization determine action to eliminate the causes of potential nonconformities in order to prevent their occurrence and are preventive actions appropriate to the effects of the potential problems?
	Has a documented procedure been established to define requirements for:
	a) Determining potential nonconformities and their causes?
	b) Evaluating the need for action to prevent occurrence of nonconformities?
	c) Determining and implementing action needed?
	d) Recording of the results of any investigations and of action taken (see 4.2.4)?
	e) Reviewing preventive action taken and its effectiveness?

Doc. Reference	Adequate?	Stage I (clauses marked *)	Stage II

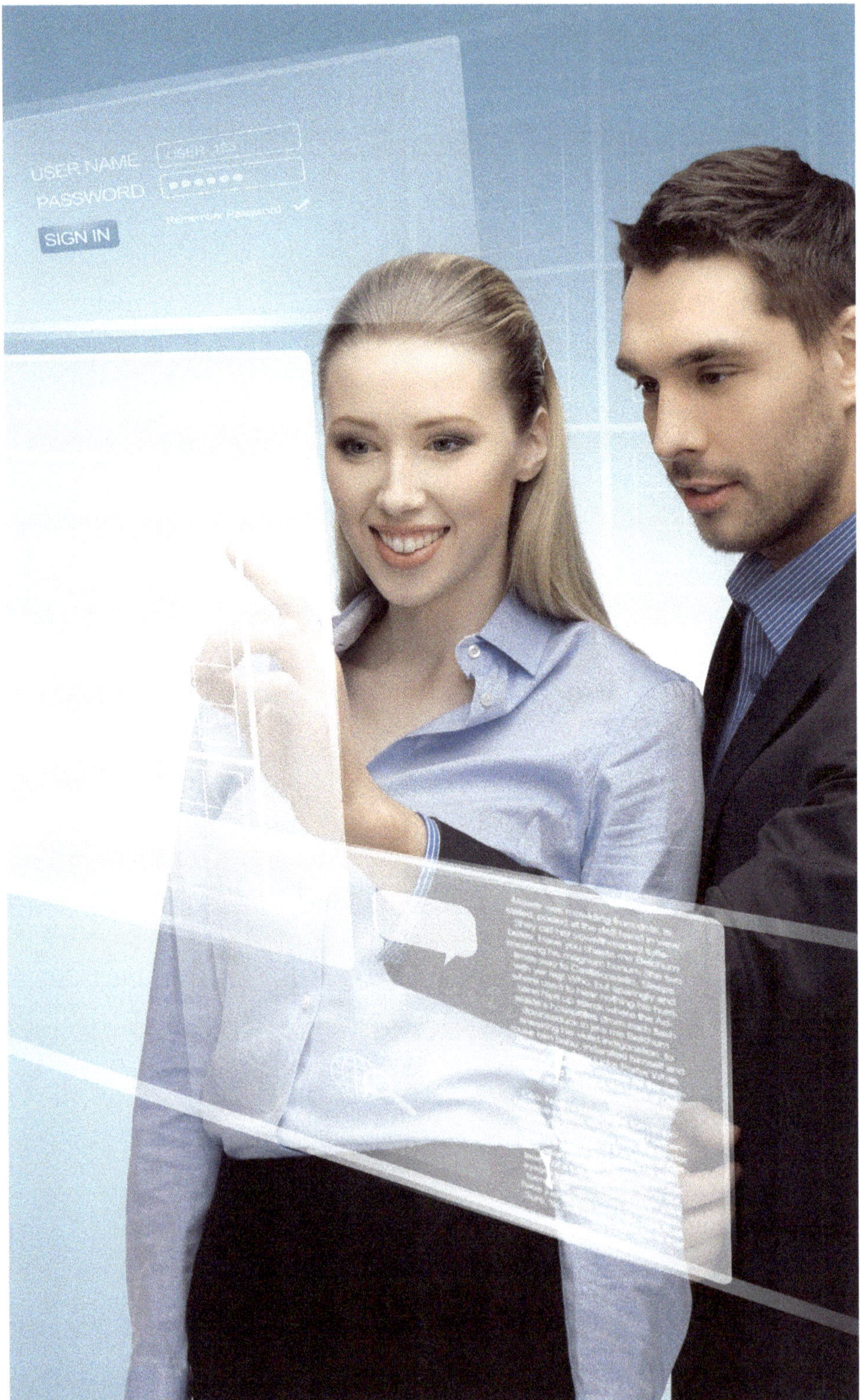
USER NAME
PASSWORD
SIGN IN

MDSAP
ISO 13485 Requirements &

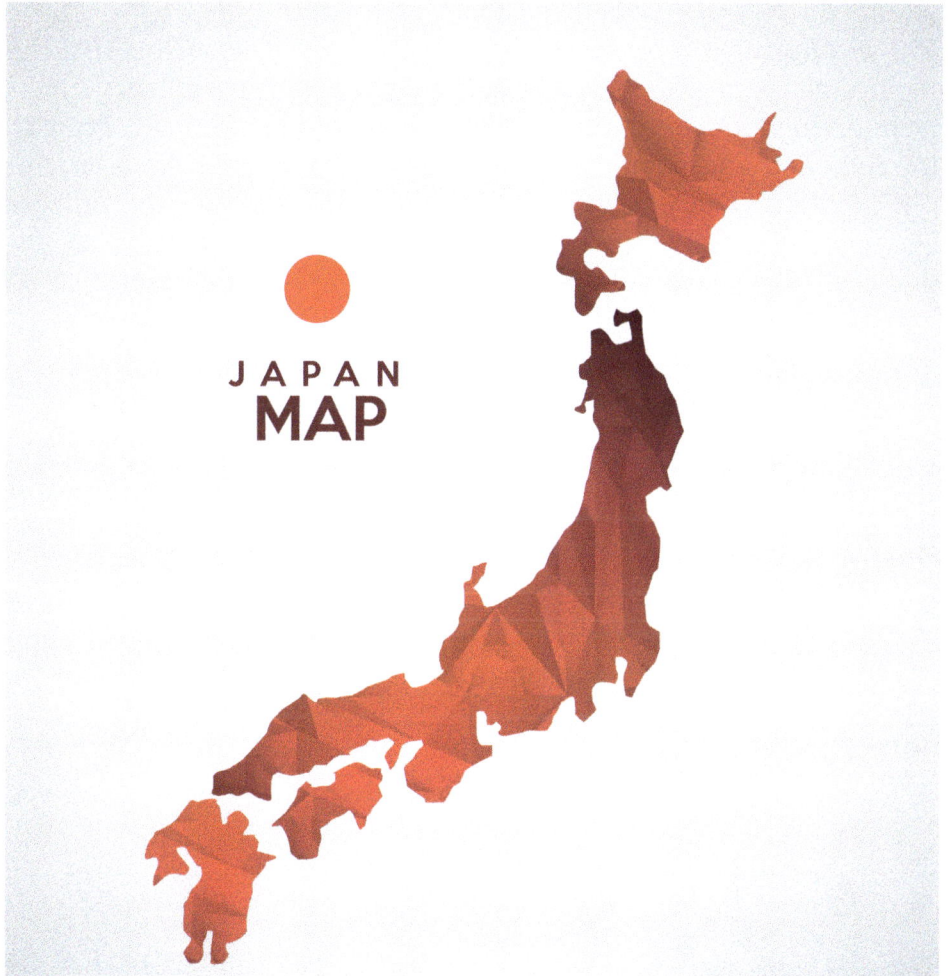

JAPAN
MAP

Management

The intent of the Management Process is to provide adequate resources for device design, manufacturing, quality assurance, distribution, installation, and servicing activities; to assure the quality management system is functioning properly and effectively; and to monitor the quality management system and make necessary adjustments. A quality management system that has been implemented effectively and is monitored to identify and address existing and potential problems is more likely to produce medical devices that function as intended.

The management representative is responsible for ensuring that the requirements of the quality management system have been effectively defined, documented, implemented, and maintained. Prior to the audit of a process, it may be helpful to interview the management representative (or designee) to obtain an overview of the process and a feel for management's knowledge and understanding of the process.

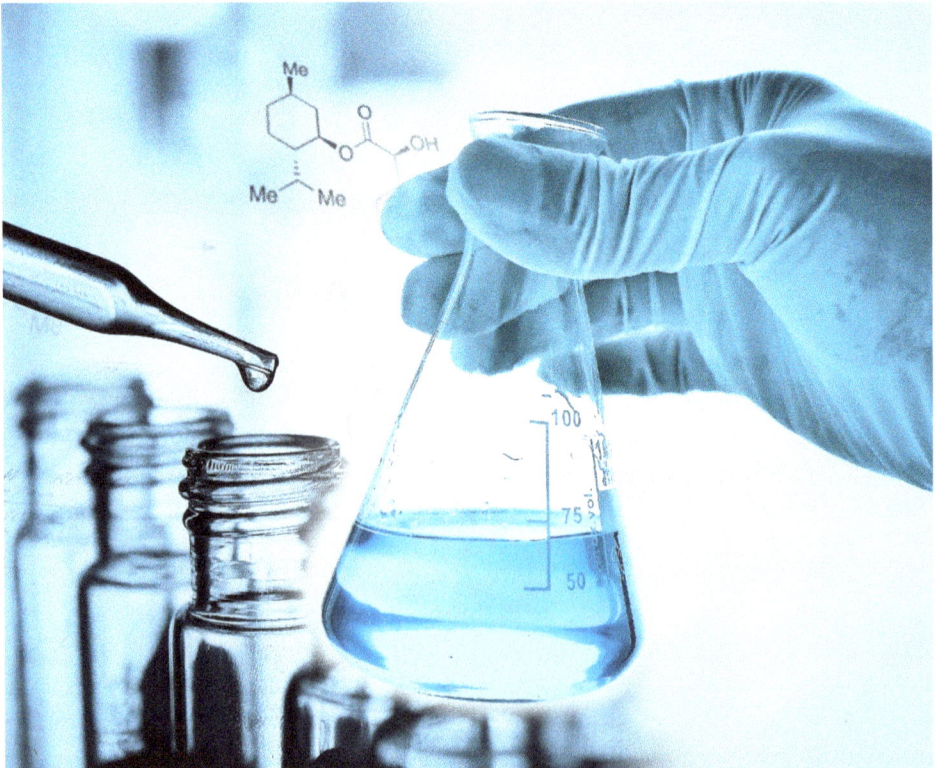

Clause and Regulation:
ISO 13485:2016: 4.1.1, 4.1.2, 4.1.3, 4.2.2, 4.1.4, 5.4.2;
MHLW/PMDA: MHLW MO169: 5, 7, 14;
MHLW/PMDA: MHLW MO169: 16, 18, 19, 20
MHLW/PMDA: MHLW MO169: 10, 15, 16, 21, 22, 23, 26

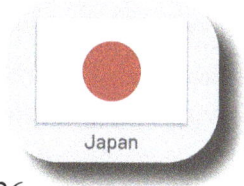
Japan

Confirm that Quality Management System documentation and records in relation to a device are retained for the following periods (5 years for training records and documentation). [MHLW MO169: 8.4, 9.3, 67, 68]. (1) 15 years for 'specially designated maintenance control required medical devices' [or one year plus the shelf life for products when the shelf life or the expiry date (hereinafter simply referred to as the "shelf life") plus one year exceeds 15 years]. (2) 5 years for the products other than the 'specially designated maintenance control required medical devices' (or one year plus the shelf life for the products of which the shelf life plus one year exceeds 5 years).

Note: The 'specially designated maintenance control required medical device' is defined as below in PMD Act 2.8:

A medical device designated by the Minister of Health, Labour and Welfare after hearing the opinion of the Pharmaceutical Affairs and Food Sanitation Council as those whose potential risk to the diagnosis, treatment or prevention of disease is significant without proper control since this kind of equipment requires expert knowledge and skill in examination for maintenance and inspection, repair and other management.

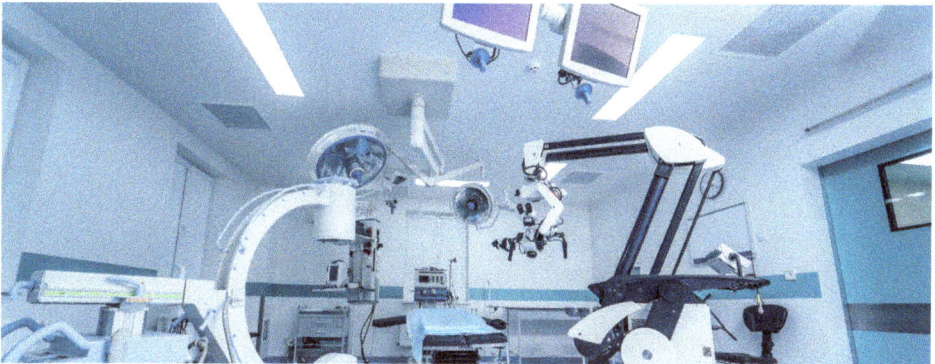

Device Marketing Authorization and Facility Registration

The Device Marketing Authorization and Facility Registration process may be audited as a linkage from the Management process and/or the Design and Development process.

ISO: ISO 13485:2016: 4.1.1, 4.2.1, 5.2, 7.2.1, 7.2.3

[PMD Act 23-2-3.1, 23-2-4]

[PMD Act 23-2-12]

Japan

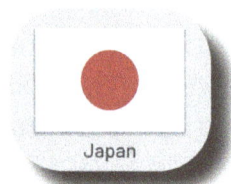

"Marketing Authorization Holder" means a person who resides in Japan and is granted a license for marketing from a prefecture government [PMD Act 23-2.1].

Application or Notification for marketing

Class 2, class 3, and class 4 medical devices except for the ones specified by the requirement of PMD Act 23-2-23.1.

An" Application for Marketing Approval" shall be submitted to PMDA by the Marketing Authorization Holder to get authorization for marketing a medical device in Japan. [PMD Act 23-2-5.1]

An "Application for QMS Audit" shall also be submitted to PMDA by the Marketing Authorization Holder, when they do not have an effective QMS Certificate for the device. [PMD Act 23-2-5.6, 7]

Class 2 and class 3 medical devices which are specified by the requirement of PMD Act 23-2-23.1

An" Application for Marketing Certification" shall be submitted to a Registered Certification Body (RCB) by the Marketing Authorization Holder to get authorization for marketing a medical device in Japan. [PMD Act 23-2-23.1].

An "Application for QMS Audit" shall also be submitted to an RCB by the person, when the person does not have a valid QMS Certificate for the device. [PMD Act 23-2-23.3, 4].

Class 1 medical device

"Notification for Marketing" shall be submitted to PMDA by the Marketing Authorization Holder for marketing a class 1 device in Japan [PMD Act 23-2-12].

A class 1 medical device doesn't need any QMS Certificate for marketing.

Facility Registration (Registered Manufacturing Site)
A medical device manufacturing site which conducts one of the designated manufacturing processes listed below shall be registered:
- Main Designing
- Main assembly
- Sterilization
- Domestic storage before final release.
The site is called "Registered Manufacturing Site". It has to submit an application to PMDA for registration by itself
[PMD Act 23-2-3.1, 23-2-4].
Any person who intends to market a medical device for business in Japan shall have a license for marketing granted by the prefectural government. This person is called a "Marketing Authorization Holder" (MAH) and shall reside in Japan [PMD Act 23-2.1]. The person has to submit an Application for Marketing Approval/Certification (class 2, 3 or 4 medical device) or a Notification for Marketing (class 1 medical device) to get marketing clearance for the medical device.
No person shall market a medical device in Japan, unless the Marketing Authorization Holder of the device has been granted the marketing clearance
[PMD Act 23-2-5.1, 23-2-23.1, 23-2-12].
A change to a medical device which is approved/certified by PMDA/a Registered Certification Body may require the Marketing Authorization Holder to submit a new application, a change application, or a change notification
[PMD Act 23-2-5.1, 23-2-5.11, 23-2-5.12, 23-2-23.1, 23-2-23.6, 23-2-23.7].
Changes that require the application or the notification are those ones which directly impact the safety and efficacy of the device and/or the substantial identity of the fact approved during marketing approval / certification.
The Registered Manufacturing Site shall communicate with the Marketing Authorization Holder about the change when the Registered Manufacturing Site plans such changes, so that the Marketing Authorization Holder could take any necessary regulatory actions mentioned above
[MHLW MO169; 29].

Examples of changes that may require an application or a notification include, but are not limited to, the following:
- Design
- Composition
- Raw material
- Sterilization method
- Manufacturing method
- Manufacturing site
- Patient or user safety features
- Operating Parameters or conditions for use
- Indication for use
- Shelf life
- Performance Specification.

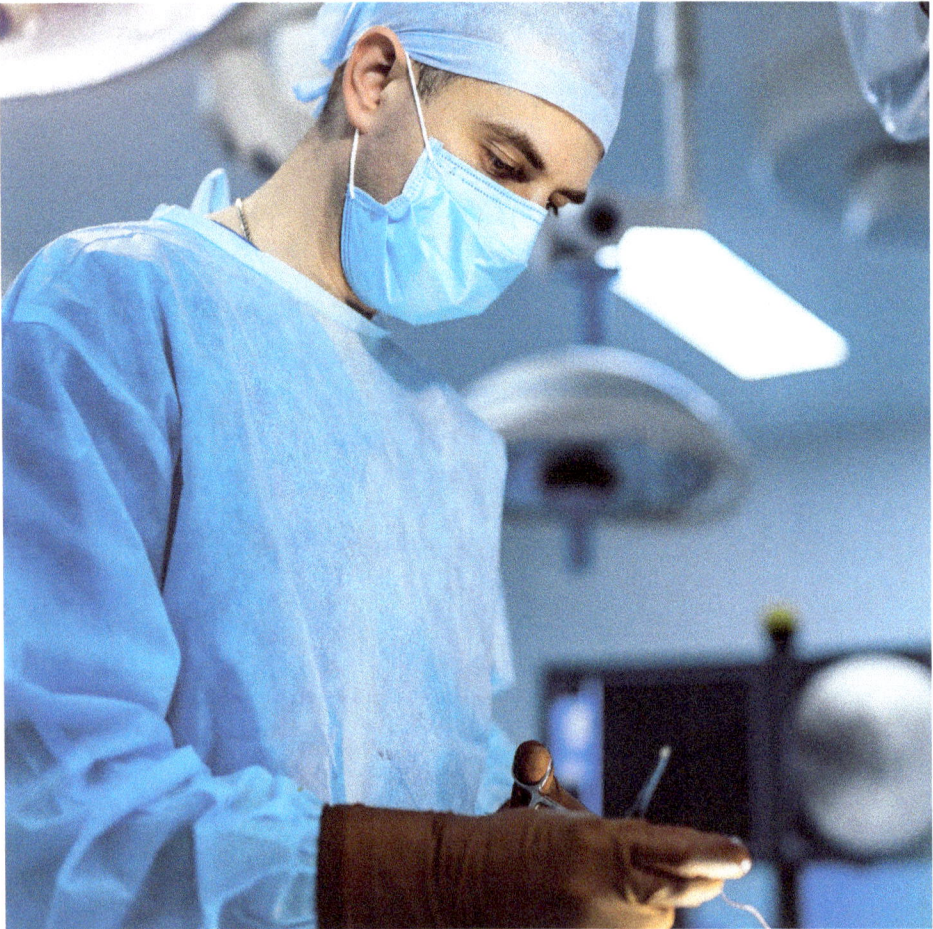

Measurement, Analysis and Improvement

One of the most important activities in the quality management system is the identification of existing and potential causes of product and quality problems. Such causes must be identified so that appropriate and effective corrective or preventive actions can take place. These activities are carried out under the Measurement, Analysis and Improvement process.

Clause and Regulation

ISO: ISO 13485:2016: 4.2.1, 8.1, 8.2.1, 8.2.6, 8.5

MHLW/PMDA: MO169: 5, 6, 54, 55, 58, 62, 63, 64

MHLW/PMDA: MO169: 37, 43, 54, 55, 58, 60, 61

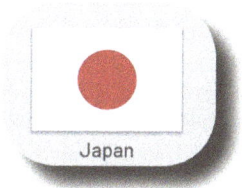

Japan

Confirm that when the Registered Manufacturing Site plans to make a significant change to a manufacturing processes (e.g. sterilization site change, manufacturing site change), the Registered Manufacturing Site notifies the Marketing Authorization Holder so as the Marketing Authorization Holder can take appropriate regulatory actions [MHLW MO169: 29].

Confirm that the person operating the Registered Manufacturing Site has determined and implemented effective arrangement for communicating with the Japanese Marketing Authorization Holder in relation to customer feedback, including customer complaints, and advisory notices [No.169: 29].

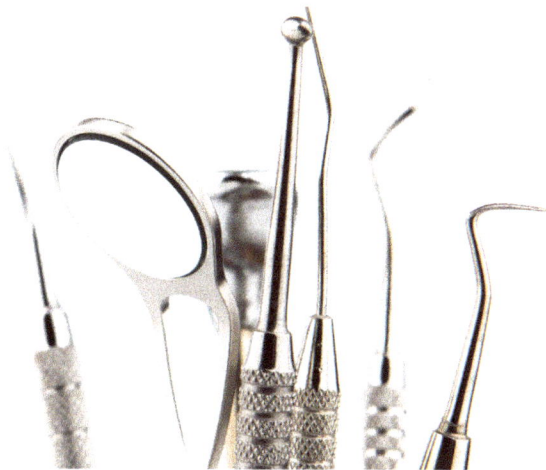

Medical Device Adverse Events and Advisory Notices Reporting
The Medical Device Adverse Events and Advisory Notices Reporting
process may be audited as a linkage from the Measurement, Analysis
and Improvement process.

Clause and Regulation
ISO: ISO 13485:2016: 4.2.1, 7.2.3, 8.2.2, 8.2.2, 8.2.3,
8.3.3
MHLW MO169: 62.6

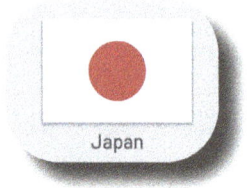

Japan

Marketing Authorization Holders are required to implement post
market safety activities in accordance with domestic (Japanese)
regulatory requirements in addition to the QMS requirements.
The persons operating the Registered Manufacturing Sites are not
required to report any adverse event directly to a Regulatory Authority, but shall report any adverse event which meets the criteria
specified by the Ordinance for Enforcement of PMD Act Article
228-20.2 to the Marketing Authorization Holder
[MHLW MO169: 62.6].
Verify that the person operating the Registered Manufacturing Site
provides events which meets the following criteria defined by the
Ordinance for Enforcement of PMD Act Article 228-20.2 (see be-
low), to the Marketing Authorization Holder in a timely manner.
- The following malfunction events which may cause or may have
caused health damage:
- Serious event (domestic and foreign)
- Unlabeled non-Serious event (domestic)
- The following Adverse Reaction events which was caused or
might have been caused by the malfunction of a medical device:
- Serious event (domestic and foreign)
- Unlabeled non-Serious event (domestic)
- Any action taken for preventing the occurrence or expansion of
public health hazard in relation to a medical device which is mar-
keted in foreign countries and is equivalent to the one marketed in
Japan. The action includes but not limited to:
- Suspension of manufacturing, importing or selling
- Recall and
- Abolishment.

- Study report that indicates:
- Possibility of event of cancer and other serious illness, injury or death caused by malfunction of a medical device (domestic and foreign), or by infectious disease arising from usage of a device (domestic and foreign)
- Significant occurrence rate change of event etc. caused by malfunction of a medical device (domestic and foreign)
- Significant occurrence rate change of infectious disease caused by usage of a medical device (domestic and foreign)
- The fact that a medical device is less effective than claimed when approved.
Marketing Authorization Holders are required to report advisory notices to Regulatory Authorities
[PMD Act 68-11].
Confirm that the person operating the Registered Manufacturing Site has determined and implemented effective arrangement for communicating with the Marketing Authorization Holder in relation to advisory notices
[MHLW MO169: 29].

Note: Persons operating Registered Manufacturing Sites are not required to report any advisory notice directly to regulatory authority, but shall communicate with the Marketing Authorization Holder, so they can take necessary regulatory actions.

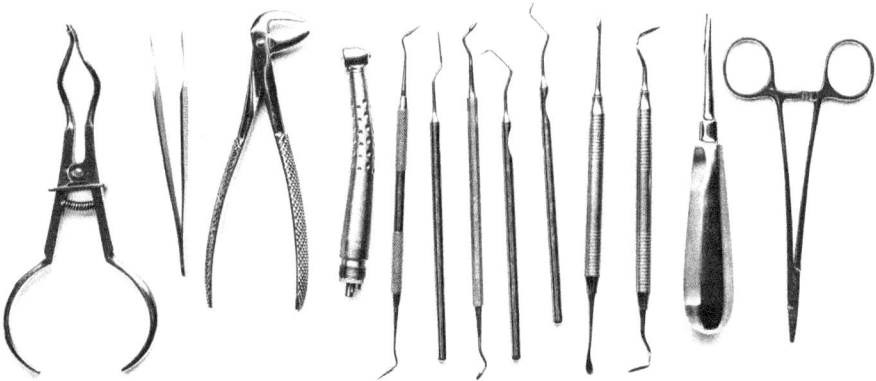

Design and Development

The purpose of the Design and Development process is to control the design of a medical device and to assure that the device meets user needs, intended use, and its specified requirements. Attention to design and development planning, identifying design inputs, developing design outputs, verifying that design outputs meet design inputs, validating the design, controlling design changes, reviewing design results, transferring the design to production, and compiling the appropriate records will help a medical device organization assure that resulting designs will meet user needs, intended uses, and requirements. Review of the Design and Development process will also provide an opportunity to evaluate how the medical device organization has utilized risk management activities to ensure design inputs are comprehensive and meet user needs, to confirm that risk control measures that were planned have been implemented in the design, and to verify that risk control measures are effective in controlling or reducing risk.

Clause and Regulation
ISO: ISO 13485:2016: 4.1.1, 4.2.1, 7.1, 7.3.10, 7.3.2
MHLW/PMDA: MO169:5, 6, 26, 30, 11, 27, 31

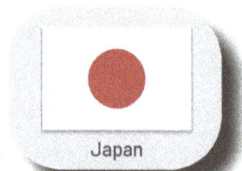

Japan

Class 1 devices are not required to comply with the requirements of MHLW MO169:30-36, which are equivalent to the requirement of design and development in ISO13485 [MHLW MO169:4.1].

For the Marketing Authorization Holder, confirm if the Marketing Authorization Holder has submitted a new application, a change application, or a change notification to PMDA/ a Registered Certification Body, when applicable [PMD Act 23-2-5.1, 23-2-5.11, 23-2-5.12, 23-2-23.1, 23-2-23.6, 23-2-23.7].

For the Registered Manufacturing Site, confirm if the site has a mechanism to communicate with the Marketing Authorization Holder about device modifications, so the Marketing Authorization Holder can take appropriate actions. If a critical medical device modification has happened in the Registered Manufacturing Site, confirm if the Registered Manufacturing Site has communicated with Marketing Authorization Holder about the change [MHLW MO169: 29].

Production and Service Controls

The purpose of the Production and Service Controls process is to manufacture products that meet specifications. Developing processes that are adequate to produce devices that meet specifications, validating (or fully verifying the results of) those processes, and monitoring and controlling those processes are all steps that help assure the result will be devices that meet specified requirements. After completing the audit of the medical device organization's Production and Service Controls process, the audit team will return to the Management process to make a final decision of whether top management ensures that an adequate and effective quality management system has been established and maintained at the medical device organization.

Clause and Regulation
ISO: ISO 13485:2016: 7.1, 7.2.1, 7.5.1, 8.2.5, 8.2.6
MHLW/PMDA: MO169: 6, 24, 25, 26, 27, 40, 41, 45, 53, 54, 57

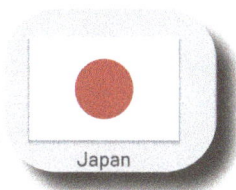

Japan

The requirements for delivery, installation, and servicing of a particular device should have already been evaluated and addressed by the medical device organization during design and development and planning for product realization.

If risk control measures were identified involving the delivery, installation, and servicing for a particular device, confirm that the necessary processes have been implemented to ensure the risk control measures are in place. For example, a medical device organization may have identified that in order for a medical imaging device to give accurate images, servicing must be performed by trained personnel according to specific instructions.

Risk control measures might include warnings on the imaging device that only authorized personnel should service the device and the design of a unique tool to access the inside of the device that is only provided to authorized service personnel.

Reviewing a validation

During review of a validation study, determine when applicable whether:

- The instruments used to generate the data were properly calibrated and maintained
- Predetermined product and process specifications were established
- Sampling plans used to collect test samples are based on a statistically valid rationale
- Data demonstrates predetermined specifications were met consistently
- Process tolerance limits were challenged
- Process equipment was properly installed, adjusted, and maintained
- Process monitoring instruments were properly calibrated and maintained
- Changes to the validated process were appropriately challenged (if applicable)
- Process operators were appropriately qualified.

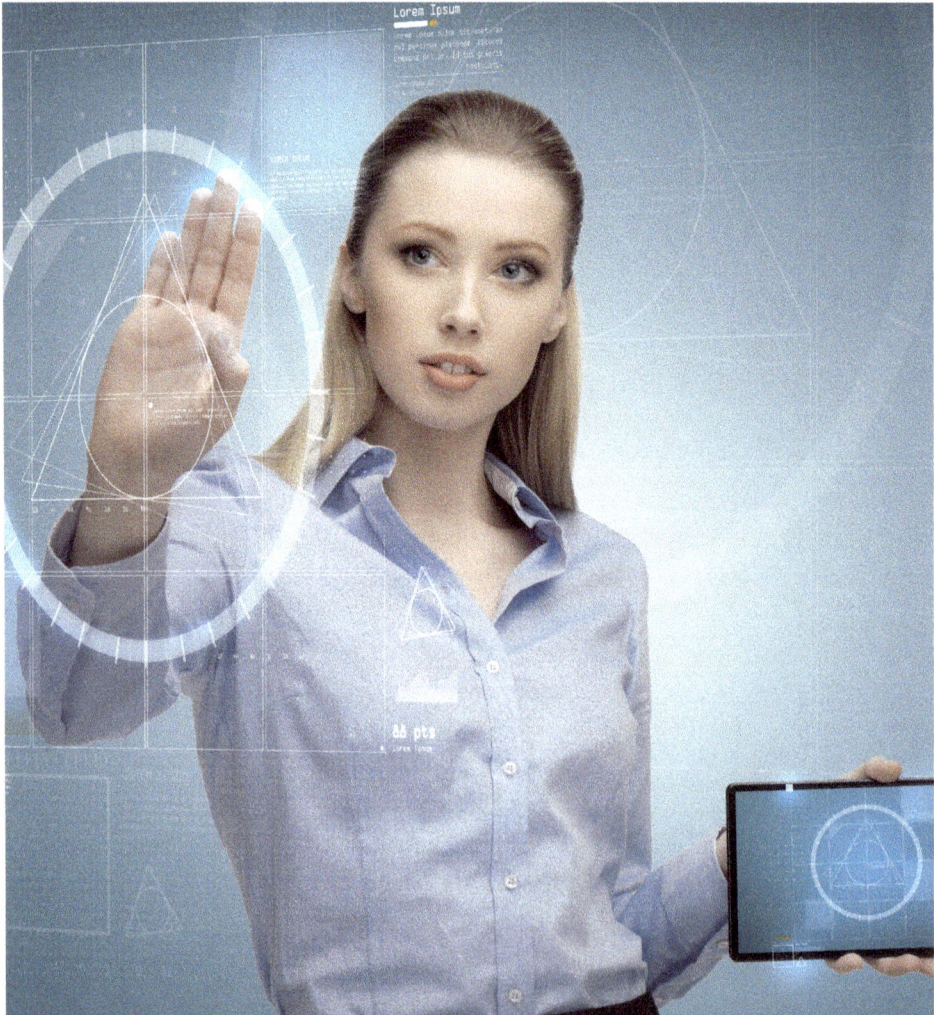

Purchasing

The intent of the Purchasing process is to ensure that purchased, sub-contracted, or otherwise received products and services conform to specified requirements. The medical device organization is expected to establish and maintain documented controls for planning and performing purchasing activities. The controls necessary depend on the effect of the product on the quality, safety, and effectiveness of the finished device. Effective purchasing processes incorporate purchasing requirements and specifications, the selection of acceptable suppliers based on the capability of the suppliers to provide acceptable product, the performance of necessary acceptance activities, and maintenance of the required quality records.

The management representative is responsible for ensuring that the requirements of the quality management system have been effectively defined, documented, implemented, and maintained. Prior to the audit of a process, it may be helpful to interview the management representative to obtain an overview of the process and a feel for management's knowledge and understanding of the process.

Clause and Regulation
ISO: ISO: ISO 13485:2016: 4.1.2, 4.1.3, 4.1.5, 7.1, 7.4.1, 7.4.2, 7.4.3

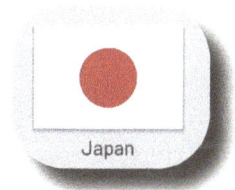

Japan

Planning

In planning product realization, the medical device organization must determine as appropriate the quality objectives and requirements for the purchased products, the processes, documents, and resources specific to the purchased products, the criteria for purchased product acceptance, and the required verification, monitoring, inspection, and test activities specific to the purchased products. Planning of product realization often begins in the design and development of the product, including the translation of the design into production specifications. The translation of the design into production specifications includes the establishment of specified requirements for purchased product.

Quality objectives

Quality objectives are typically expressed as a measurable target or goal. The planning of product realization should include consideration of how the purchased product, the criteria for purchased product acceptance, and the required verification, monitoring, inspection, and test activities specific to the purchased product will achieve the quality objectives.

- Some examples of QOB include:
- Number of complaints -v- number of parts shipped
- On-time delivery %
- Supplier parts rejected
- Comparison of internal audit findings -v- external audit findings
- Achieving a certain accuracy if you're developing product - based software
- Annual Post-market surveillance
- Auditing our system for regulatory compliance

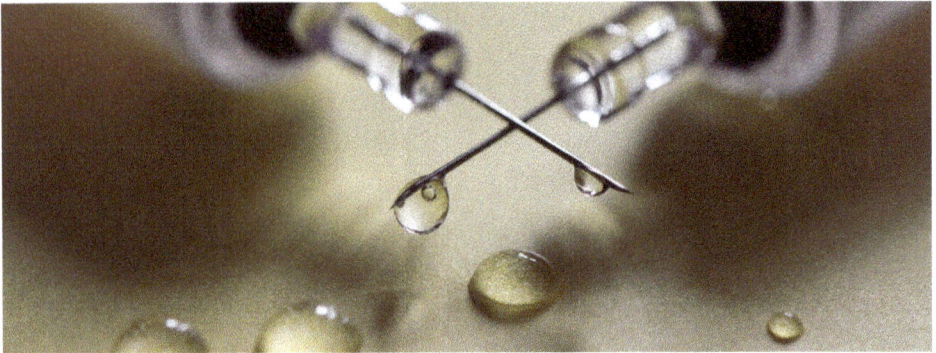

Some managers believe that the reward for hard work should be a paycheck. That's sort of like telling your children that they get to eat for doing something you're proud of. Employees are not children, but you are responsible for developing them into more valuable employees so that they can be promoted. If there is no incentive, your team will not be engaged. Therefore, pick a reward that is proportional to the bottom-line impact. Five percent of the bottom-line impact is what I like to target, but you would be amazed at how effective a few small rewards at each milestone can be. If you have trouble getting management approval for rewards, remind your boss of the bottom-line impact and link the rewards closely to the impact.

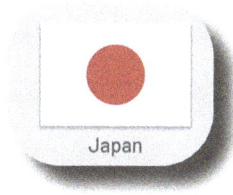

Japan

MDSAP
Audit Checklist

	REQUIREMENTS
4 Quality management system	
4.1 General requirements	
	Has the organization:
	a) identified the processes needed for the quality management system and their application throughout the organization (see 1.2)?
	b) determined the sequence and interaction of these processes?
	c) determined criteria and methods needed to ensure that both the operation and control of these processes are effective?
	d) ensured the availability of resources and information necessary to support the operation and monitoring of their processes?
	e) monitored, measured, and analyzed these processes
	f) implemented actions necessary to achieve planned results and maintain the effectiveness of these processes?
	Does the organization manage these processes in accordance with the requirements of this International Standard?
	Where an organization chooses to outsource any process that affects product conformity with requirements, does the organization ensure control over such processes?
	Is the control of such outsourced processes identified within the quality management system? (see 8.5.1)
4.2.1 General	

Doc. Reference	Adequate?	Stage I (clauses marked *)	Stage II
	Y/N	Initial›s	Initial›s

	REQUIREMENTS
	Does the quality management system documentation include:
	a) documented statements of a quality policy and quality objectives?
	b) a quality manual?
	c) documented procedures required by this international standard?
	d) documents needed by the organization to ensure the effective planning, operation and control of its processes?
	e) records required by this International Standard (see 4.2.4)?
	f) any other documentation specified by national or regional regulations?
	Has the organization established and maintained a file for each type or model of medical device either containing or identifying documents defining product specifications and quality system requirements (see 4.2.3)?
	Do these documents define the complete manufacturing process and, if applicable, installation and servicing?
EU	Does the file contain or refer to the location of objective evidence establishing the safety and effectiveness of the device as required by Annex 1 of the MDD? (MDD Annex I)
4.2.2 Quality manual	
	Has the organization established and maintained a quality manual that includes:
	a) the scope of the quality management system, including details of and justification for any exclusion and/or non-application (see 1.2)?
	b) the documented procedures established for the quality management system, or reference to them?
	c) a description of the interaction between the processes of the quality management system?

Doc. Reference	Adequate?	Stage I (clauses marked *)	Stage II

	REQUIREMENTS	
	Does the quality manual outline the structure of the documentation used in the quality management system?	
Japan	Confirm that the products distributed in the Japanese market, are approved/ certified/ notified with PMDA/ Registered Certification Bodies [PMD Act: -2-23 ,(1) 5-2-23 1) 12-2-23 ,(1) 23)]. For a manufacturing site which conducts primary design, primary assembly, sterilization, domestic storage until final release of products, confirm that the site is registered by MHLW. [PMD Act: 4-2-23 ,3-2-23]	
EU	Are the applicable sections of the Medical Device Directive (MDD) included in the specified requirements throughout the documented quality system? Interpretation: A statement only indicating compliance/conformity with the relevant international or EU regulatory requirements is not acceptable.	
4.2.3 Control of documents		
	Are documents required by the quality management system controlled?	

Doc. Reference	Adequate?	Stage I (clauses marked *)	Stage II

	REQUIREMENTS
	Is a documented procedure established to define the controls needed:
	a) To review and approve documents for adequacy prior to issue?
	b) To review and update as necessary and re-approve documents?
	c) To ensure that changes and the current revision status of documents are identified?
	d) To ensure that relevant versions of applicable documents are available at points of use?
	e) To ensure the documents remain legible and readily identifiable?
	f) To ensure that documents of external origin are identified and their distribution controlled?
	g) To prevent the unintended use of obsolete documents and to apply suitable identification to them if they are retained for any purpose?
	Does the organization ensure that changes to documents are reviewed and approved either by the original approving function or another designated function which has access to pertinent background information upon which to base its decisions?
	Does the organization define the period for which at least one copy of obsolete controlled documents shall be retained?
	Does this period ensure that documents to which medical devices have been manufactured and tested are available for at least the lifetime of the medical device as defined by the organization, but not less than the retention period of any resulting record (see 4.2.4), or as specified by relevant regulatory requirements?

Doc. Reference	Adequate?	Stage I (clauses marked *)	Stage II

	REQUIREMENTS
Japan	Confirm that Quality Management System documentation and records in relation to a device are retained by the Registered Manufacturing Site for the following periods [MHLW Ministerial Ordinance No.9.3 ,8.4 :169, 68 ,67]: 15 .1 years for "specially designated maintenance control required medical devices" [or one year plus the shelf life for products when the shelf life or the expiry date (hereinafter simply referred to as the «shelf life») plus one year exceeds 15 years] 5 .2 years for the products other than the 'specially designated maintenance control required medical devices' (or one year plus the shelf life for the products of which the shelf life plus one year exceeds 5 years). 5 .3 years for training records and documentation Note: PMD Act 2.8 defines the term "specially designated maintenance control required medical device" as: A medical device designated by the Minister of Health, Labour and Welfare after hearing the opinion of the Pharmaceutical Affairs and Food Sanitation Council as those whose potential risk to the diagnosis, treatment or prevention of disease is significant without proper control since this kind of equipment requires expert knowledge and skill in examination for maintenance and inspection, repair and other management.
	4.2.4 Control of quality records

Doc. Reference	Adequate?	Stage I (clauses marked *)	Stage II

	REQUIREMENTS	
	Are records established and maintained to provide evidence of conformity to requirements and of the effective operation of the quality management system?	
	Do records remain legible, readily identifiable and retrievable?	
	Has a documented procedure been established to define the controls needed for the identification, storage, protection, retrieval, retention time and disposition of records?	
	Does the organization retain the records for a period of time at least equivalent to the lifetime of the medical device as defined by the organization, but not less than two years from the date of product release by the organization or as specified by relevant regulatory requirements?	
EU	Has the manufacturer retained for a period ending at least five years after the last product has been manufactured, the records listed in Annex II, 6.1 or Annex V, 5.1 or Annex VI, 5.1 (whichever applies)	
5 Management responsibility		
5.1 Management commitment		
	Has top management provided evidence of its commitment to the development and implementation of the quality management system and maintaining its effectiveness by:	
	a) Communicating to the organization the importance of meeting customer as well as statutory and regulatory requirements?	
	b) Establishing the quality policy?	
	c) Ensuring that quality objectives are established?	
	d) Conducting management reviews?	
	e) Ensuring the availability of resources?	
5.2 Customer focus		
	Does top management ensure that customer requirements are determined and met (see 7.2.1 and 8.2.1)?	

Doc. Reference	Adequate?	Stage I (clauses marked *)	Stage II

	REQUIREMENTS
	5.3 Quality policy
	Does top management ensure that the quality policy
	a) Is appropriate to the purpose of the organization?
	b) Includes a commitment to comply with requirements and to maintain the effectiveness of the quality management system?
	c) Provides a framework for establishing and reviewing quality objectives?
	d) Is communicated and understood within the organization?
	e) Is reviewed for continuing suitability?
5.4 Planning	
5.4.1 Quality objectives	
	Does top management ensure that quality objectives, including those needed to meet requirements for product (see 7.1a), are established at relevant functions and levels within the organization?
	Are quality objectives measurable?
	Are quality objectives consistent with the quality policy?
5.4.2 Quality management system planning	
	Has top management ensured that:
	a) The planning of the quality management system is carried out in order to meet the requirements given in 4.1, as well as the quality objectives?
	b) The integrity of the quality management system is maintained when changes to the quality management system are planned and implemented?
5.5 Responsibility, authority and communication	
5.5.1 Responsibility and authority	

Doc. Reference	Adequate?	Stage I (clauses marked *)	Stage II

	REQUIREMENTS
	Has top management ensured that responsibilities and authorities were defined, documented and communicated within the organization?
	Has top management established the interrelation of all personnel who manage, perform and verify work affecting quality, and ensured the independence and authority necessary to perform these tasks?
5.5.2 Management representative	
	Has top management appointed a member of management who, irrespective of other responsibilities, has responsibility and authority that includes:
	a) Ensuring that processes needed for the quality management system are established, implemented, and maintained?
	b) Reporting to top management on the performance of the quality management system and any need for improvement (see 8.5)?
	c) Ensuring the promotion of awareness of regulatory and customer requirements throughout the organization?
5.5.3 Internal communication	
	Has top management ensured that appropriate communication processes have been established within the organization and that communication takes place regarding the effectiveness of the quality management system?
5.6 Management review	
5.6.1 General	
	Does top management review the organization's quality management system, at planned intervals, to ensure its continuing suitability, adequacy and effectiveness?

Doc. Reference	Adequate?	Stage I (clauses marked *)	Stage II

	REQUIREMENTS	
	Does this review include assessing opportunities for improvement and the need for changes to the quality management system, including the quality policy and quality objectives?	
	Are records from management reviews maintained (see 4.2.4)?	
5.6.2 Review input		
	Does the input to management review include information on:	
	a) Results of audits?	
	b) Customer feedback?	
	c) Process performance and product conformity?	
	d) Status of preventive and corrective actions?	
	e) Follow-up actions from previous management reviews?	
	f) Changes that could affect the quality management system?	
	g) Recommendations for improvement?	
	h) New or revised regulatory requirements?	
5.6.3 Review output		
	Does output from the management review include any decisions and actions related to:	
	a) Improvements needed to maintain the effectiveness of the quality management system and its processes?	
	b) Improvement of product related to customer requirements?	
	c) Resource needs?	
6 Resource management		
6.1 Provision of resources		

Doc. Reference	Adequate?	Stage I (clauses marked *)	Stage II

	REQUIREMENTS
	Does the organization determine and provide the resources needed:
	a) To implement the quality management system and to maintain its effectiveness?
	b) To meet regulatory and customer requirements?
6.2 Human resources	
6.2.1 General	
	Are personnel performing work affecting product quality competent on the basis of appropriate education, training, skills and experience?
6.2.2 Competence, awareness and training	
	Does the organization:
	a) determine the necessary competence for personnel performing work affecting product quality?
	b) Provide training or take other actions to satisfy these needs?
	c) Evaluate the effectiveness of actions taken?
	d) Ensure that its personnel are aware of the relevance and importance of their activities and how they contribute to the achievement of the quality objectives?
	e) Maintain appropriate records of education, training, skills and experience (see 4.2.4)?
6.3 Infrastructure	
	Does the organization determine, provide and maintain the infrastructure needed to achieve conformity to product requirements?
	Infrastructure includes, as applicable:
	a) Buildings, workspace and associated utilities
	b) Process equipment, both hardware and software
	c) Supporting services such as transport or communication

Doc. Reference	Adequate?	Stage I (clauses marked *)	Stage II

	REQUIREMENTS
	Does the organization establish documented requirements for maintenance activities, including their frequency, when such activities or lack thereof can affect product quality?
	Are records of such maintenance maintained (see 4.2.4)?
	Has the organization determined and does it manage the work environment needed to achieve conformity to product requirements?
	a) Has the organization established documented requirements for health, cleanliness and clothing of personnel if contact between such personnel and the product or work environment could adversely affect the quality of the product (see 7.5.1.2.1)?
	b) If work environment conditions can have an adverse effect on product quality, has organization established documented requirements for the work environment conditions and documented procedures or work instructions to monitor and control these work environment conditions (see 7.5.1.2.1)?
	c) Does the organization ensure that all personnel who are required to work temporarily under special environmental conditions within the work environment are appropriately trained or supervised by a trained person [see 6.2.2 b)]?
	d) If appropriate, are special arrangements established and documented for the control of contaminated or potentially contaminated product in order to prevent contamination of other product, the work environment or personnel (see 7.5.3.1)?
7 Product realization	
7.1 Planning of product realization	
	Has the organization planned and developed the processes needed for product realization?

Doc. Reference	Adequate?	Stage I (clauses marked *)	Stage II

	REQUIREMENTS
	Is the planning of product realization consistent with the requirements of the other processes of the quality management system (see 4.1)?
	In planning product realization, has the organization determined the following, as appropriate:
	a) Quality objectives and requirements for products?
	b) The need to establish processes, documents, and provide resources specific to the product?
	c) Required verification, validation, monitoring, inspection and test activities specific to the product and the criteria for product acceptance?
	d) Records needed to provide evidence that the realization processes and resulting product meet requirements (see 4.2.4)?
	Is the output of this planning in a form suitable for the organization's method of operations?
	Does the organization establish documented requirements for risk management throughout product realization and are records arising from risk management maintained (see 4.2.4)?
EU	Does the supplier evaluate the need for risk analysis throughout the design process and maintain records of any risk analysis performed? (MDD Annex 1)

7.2.1 Determination of requirements related to the product

Doc. Reference	Adequate?	Stage I (clauses marked *)	Stage II

		REQUIREMENTS
		Has the organization determined:
		a) Requirements specified by the customer, including the requirements for delivery and post-delivery activities?
		b) Requirements not stated by the customer but necessary for specified or intended use, where known?
		c) Statutory and regulatory requirements related to the product?
		d) Any additional requirements determined by the organization?
	EU	Vefiy that manufacturing maintains files containing or refer to the location of objective evidence establishing the safety and effectiveness of the device as required by Annex 1 of the MDD. Verify that the manufacturer followed a defined and effective process to establish and maintain a file containing documents defining product specifications and quality system requirements for each newa and existing type/modes of medical devices. Since the last audit, has the manufacturer introduced new products in the EU? Has the manufacturer followed a defined and effective process to obtain an approval from the Notified Body to CE mark a product prior to selling it in the EU? (does not apply to class I devices)

Doc. Reference	Adequate?	Stage I (clauses marked *)	Stage II

	REQUIREMENTS
Japan	Verify that that a «Application for Marketing Approval» or « Notification for Marketing» has been submitted by the MAH; and that the manufacturing facility has been registered. 1) Class 2, class 3, and class 4 medical devices except for the devices specified by the requirement of PMD Act: 223-23 (1): An "Application for Marketing Approval" shall be submitted to PMDA by the Marketing Authorization Holder to receive authorization for marketing a medical device in Japan. [PMD Act: 1) 5-2-23)] An "Application for QMS Audit" shall also be submitted to PMDA by the Marketing Authorization Holder, when they do not have an effective QMS Certificate for the device. [PMD Act: 5-2-23 7) ,(6))] 2) Class 2 and class 3 medical devices which are specified by the requirement of PMD Act: 1) 23-2-23): An "Application for Marketing Certification" shall be submitted to a Registered Certification Body (RCB) by the Marketing Authorization Holder to receive authorization for marketing a medical device in Japan. [PMD Act: 1) 23-2-23)] An "Application for QMS Audit" shall also be submitted to an RCB by the person, when the person does not have a valid QMS Certificate for the device. [PMD Act: 4) ,(3) 23-2-23)]. Facility Registration (Registered Manufacturing Site): A medical device manufacturing site which conducts one of the designated manufacturing processes listed below shall be registered: a) Primary Designing, b) Primary assembly, c) Sterilization, and
	7.2.2 Review of requirements related to the product

Doc. Reference	Adequate?	Stage I (clauses marked *)	Stage II

	REQUIREMENTS
	Does the organization review the requirements related to the product?
	Is this review conducted prior to the organization's commitment to supply a product to the customer (e.g. submission of tenders, acceptance of contracts or orders, acceptance of changes to contracts or orders)?
	Does the organization ensure that:
	a) Product requirements are defined and documented?
	b) Contract or order requirements differing from those previously expressed are resolved?
	c) The organization has the ability to meet the defined requirements?
	Are records of the results of the review and actions arising from the review maintained (see 4.2.4)?
	Where the customer provides no documented statement of requirement, are the customer requirements confirmed by the organization before acceptance?
	Where product requirements are changed, does the organization ensure that relevant documents are amended and that relevant personnel are made aware of the changed requirements?
7.2.3 Customer communication	
	Has the organization determined and implemented effective arrangements for communicating with customers in relation to:
	a) Product information?
	b) Enquiries, contracts or order handling, including amendments?
	c) Customer feedback, including customer complaints? (see 8.2.1)
	d) Advisory notices? (see 8.5.1)
7.3 Design and development	

Doc. Reference	Adequate?	Stage I (clauses marked *)	Stage II

	REQUIREMENTS

7.3.1 Design and/or development planning	
	Has the organization established documented procedures for design and development?
	Does the organization plan and control the design and development of product?
	During the design and development planning, does the organization determine:
	a) The design and development stages?
	b) The review, verification, validation and design transfer activities (see Note) that are appropriate at each design and development stage?
	c) The responsibilities and authorities for design and development?
	Does the organization manage the interfaces between different groups involved in design and development to ensure effective communication and clear assignment of responsibility?
	Is planning output documented, and updated as appropriate, as the design and development progresses? (See 4.2.3)
7.3.2 Design and development inputs	
	Have inputs relating to product requirements been determined and records maintained (see 4.2.4)?
	Do these inputs include:
	a) Functional, performance and safety requirements, according to the intended use?
	b) Applicable statutory and regulatory requirements?
	c) Where applicable, information derived from previous similar designs?
	d) Other requirements essential for design and development?
	e) Output(s) of risk management (see 7.1)?

Doc. Reference	Adequate?	Stage I (clauses marked *)	Stage II

	REQUIREMENTS
	Are these inputs reviewed for adequacy and approved?
	Are requirements complete, unambiguous and not in conflict with each other?
7.3.3 Design and development outputs	
	Are the outputs of design and development provided in a form that enables verification against the design and development input, and is it approved prior to release?
	Do design and development outputs:
	a) meet the input requirements for design and development?
	b) Provide appropriate information for purchasing, production and for service provision?
	c) Contain or reference product acceptance criteria?
	d) Specify the characteristics of the product that are essential for its safe and proper use?
	Are records of the design and development outputs maintained (see 4.2.4)?
7.3.4 Design and development review	
	At suitable stages, are systematic reviews of design and development performed in accordance with planned arrangements (see 7.3.1):
	a) To evaluate the ability of the results of design and development to meet requirements?
	b) To identify any problems and propose necessary actions?
	Do participants in such reviews include representatives of functions concerned with the design and development stage(s) being reviewed, as well as other specialist personnel (see 5.5.1 and 6.2.1)?
	Are records of the results of the reviews and any necessary actions maintained (see 4.2.4)?
EU	Does the supplier evaluate the need for risk analysis throughout the design process and maintain records of any risk analysis performed? (MDD Annex 1)

Doc. Reference	Adequate?	Stage I (clauses marked *)	Stage II

	REQUIREMENTS

7.3.5 Design and development verification	
	Is verification performed in accordance with planned arrangements (see 7.3.1) to ensure that the design and development outputs have met the design and development input requirements?
	Are records of the results of the verification and any necessary actions maintained?
7.3.6 Design and development validation	
	Is design and development validation performed in accordance with planned arrangements (see 7.3.1) to ensure that the resulting product is capable of meeting the requirements for the specified application or intended use?
	Is validation completed prior to the delivery or implementation of the product (see Note 1)?
	Are records of the results of validation and any necessary actions maintained (see 4.2.4)?
	As part of design and development validation, does the organization perform clinical evaluations and/or evaluation of performance of the medical device, as required by national or regional regulations (see Note 2)?
7.3.7 Control of design and development changes	
	Are design and development changes identified and records maintained?
	Are changes reviewed, verified, and validated, as appropriate, and approved before implementation?
	Does the review of design and development changes include evaluation of the effect of the changes on constituent parts and product already delivered?
	Are records of the results of the review of changes and any necessary actions maintained?

Doc. Reference	Adequate?	Stage I (clauses marked *)	Stage II

	REQUIREMENTS
Japan	For the Marketing Authorization Holder: When applicable, confirm the Marketing Authorization Holder has submitted a new application, a change application, or a change notification to PMDA/ a Registered Certification Body. For the Registered Manufacturing Site: Confirm the site has a mechanism to communicate with the Marketing Authorization Holder about device modifications so the Marketing Authorization Holder can take appropriate actions when necessary. If a critical medical device modification has occurred at the Registered Manufacturing Site, confirm if the Registered Manufacturing Site has communicated the change to the Marketing Authorization Holder. A change to a medical device which is approved/certified by PMDA/a Registered Certification Body marequire the Marketing Authorization Holder to submit a change application or a change notification [PMDAct ,(1) 5-2-23 23-2-23 ,(6) 23-2-23 ,(1) 23-2-23 ,(12) 5-2-23 ,(11) 5-2-23 7))]. Changes that require a change application or a change notification are those which directly impact the safety and efficacy of thdevice; and/or the intended use, materials, etc. approved during marketing approval / certification. The Registered Manufacturing Site shall communicate changes with the Marketing Authorization Holder when the Registered Manufacturing Site plans such changes. This allows the Marketing AuthorizationHolder to take any necessary regulatory actions mentioned above [MHLW MO29 ;169]. Examples of changes that may require an application or a notification include, but are not limited to: • Design; Composition; Raw material; Sterilization method; • Manufacturing method; Manufacturing site; Patient or user safety features; Operating parameters or conditions for use; Indication for use; Shelf life; Performance specification.

Doc. Reference	Adequate?	Stage I (clauses marked *)	Stage II

	REQUIREMENTS
EU	Do documented procedures identify the need to report essential changes to the Notified Body, (MDD Annex II, V, VI, 3.4)
7.4 Purchasing	
7.4.1 Purchasing process	
	Has the organization established documented procedures to ensure that purchased product conforms to specified purchase requirements?
	Is the type and extent of control applied to the supplier and the purchased product dependent upon the effect of the purchased product on subsequent product realization or the final product?
	Does the organization evaluate and select suppliers based on their ability to supply product in accordance with the organization's requirements?
	Have criteria for selection, evaluation and re-evaluation been established?
	Are records of the results of evaluation and any necessary actions arising from the evaluation maintained (see 4.2.4)?

Doc. Reference	Adequate?	Stage I (clauses marked *)	Stage II

	REQUIREMENTS
Japan	For Marketing Authorization Holder: If the Marketing Authorization Holder (MAH) has outsourced to a Registered Manufacturing Site (RMS) any process that affects product conformity with requirements, verify the MAH has performed the necessary verification that the RMS has an appropriate quality management system. If the site of a supplier is a Registered Manufacturing Site, verify the MAH has performed the necessary verification that the supplier has an appropriate qualitymanagement system [MHLW MO65 :169].
	For Registered Manufacturing Sites: If the RMS has outsourced to another RMS any process that affects product conformity with requirements, confirm the outsourcing RMS has performed the necessary verification that the outsourced RMS has an appropriate quality management system. If the site of a supplier is an RMS, verify the purchase controlling RMS has performed the necessary verification that the supplier has an appropriate quality management system [MHLW MO65 :169].
7.4.2 Purchasing information	
	Does purchasing information describe the product to be purchased, including where appropriate:
	a) Requirements for approval of product, procedures, processes and equipment?
	b) Requirements for qualification of personnel?
	c) Quality management system requirements?
	Does the organization ensure the adequacy of specified purchase requirements prior to their communication to the supplier?
	To the extent required for traceability given in 7.5.3.2, does the organization maintain relevant purchasing information, i.e. documents (see 4.2.3) and records (see 4.2.4)?

Doc. Reference	Adequate?	Stage I (clauses marked *)	Stage II

	REQUIREMENTS
7.4.3 Verification of purchased product	
	Has the organization established and implemented the inspection or other activities necessary for ensuring that purchased product meets specified purchase requirements?
	Where the organization or its customer intends to perform verification at the supplier's premises, does the organization state the intended verification arrangements and method of product release in the purchasing information?
	Are records of the verification maintained (see 4.2.4)?
7.5 Production and service provision	
7.5.1 Control of production and service provision	
7.5.1.1 General Requirements	
	Does the organization plan and carry out production and service provision under controlled conditions?
	Do the controlled conditions include, as applicable:
	a) The availability of information that describes the characteristics of the product?
	b) The availability of documented procedures, documented requirements, work instructions, reference materials and reference measurement procedures as necessary?
	c) The use of suitable equipment?
	d) The availability and use of monitoring and measuring devices?
	e) The implementation of monitoring and measurement?
	f) The implementation of release, delivery and post-delivery activities?
	g) The implementation of defined operations for labeling and packaging?

Doc. Reference	Adequate?	Stage I (clauses marked *)	Stage II

	REQUIREMENTS
	Does the organization establish and maintain a record (see 4.2.4) for each batch of medical devices that provides traceability to the extent specified in 7.5.3 and identifies the amount manufactured and amount approved for distribution?
	Is the batch record verified and approved?

7.5.1.2 Control of production and service provision — Specific requirement

7.5.1.2.1 Cleanliness of product and contamination control

	Does the organization establish documented requirements for cleanliness of product if:
	a) Product is cleaned by the organization prior to sterilization and/or its use, or
	b) Product is supplied non-sterile to be subjected to a cleaning process prior to sterilization and/or its use, or
	c) Product is supplied to be used non-sterile and its cleanliness is of significance in use, or
	d) Process agents are to be removed from product during manufacture?
	If product is cleaned in accordance with a) or b) above, the requirements contained in 6.4 a) and 6.4 b) do not apply prior to the cleaning process.

7.5.1.2.2 Installation activities

	If appropriate, does the organization establish documented requirements which contain acceptance criteria for installing and verifying the installation of the medical device?
	If the agreed customer requirements allow installation to be performed other than by the organization or its authorized agent, does the organization provide documented requirements for installation and verification?
	Are records of installation and verification performed by the organization or its authorized agent maintained (see 4.2.4)?

Doc. Reference	Adequate?	Stage I (clauses marked *)	Stage II

	REQUIREMENTS	

7.5.1.2.3 Servicing activities		
	If servicing is a specified requirement, does the organization establish documented procedures, work instructions and reference materials and reference measurement procedures, as necessary, for performing servicing activities and verifying that they meet the specified requirements?	
	Are records of servicing activities carried out by the organization maintained (see 4.2.4)?	

7.5.1.3 Particular requirements for sterile medical devices		
	Does the organization maintain records of the process parameters for the sterilization process which was used for each sterilization batch (see 4.2.4)?	
	Are sterilization records traceable to each production batch of medical devices (see 7.5.1.1)?	

7.5.2 Validation of processes for production and service provision		

7.5.2.1 General requirements		
	Does the organization validate any processes for production and service provision where the resulting output cannot be verified by subsequent monitoring or measurement? (this includes any processes where deficiencies become apparent only after the product is in use or the service has been delivered)	
	Does validation demonstrate the ability of the processes to achieve planned results?	
	Has the organization established arrangements for these processes including, as applicable:	
	a) Defined criteria for review and approval of the processes?	
	b) Approval of equipment and qualification of personnel?	
	c) Use of specific methods and procedures?	
	d) Requirements for records (see 4.2.4)?	
	e) Re-validation?	

Doc. Reference	Adequate?	Stage I (clauses marked *)	Stage II

	REQUIREMENTS
	Has the organization established documented procedures for the validation of the application of computer software (and changes to such software and/or its application) for production and service provision that affect the ability of the product to conform to specified requirements?
	Are such software applications validated prior to initial use?
	Are records of validation maintained (see 4.2.4)?
7.5.2.2 Particular requirements for sterile medical devices	
	Has the organization established documented procedures for the validation of sterilization processes?
	Are sterilization processes validated prior to initial use?
	Are records of validation of each sterilization process maintained (see 4.2.4)?
7.5.3 Identification and traceability	
7.5.3.1 Identification	
	Does the organization identify the product by suitable means throughout product realization and does the organization establish documented procedures for such product identification?
	Has the organization established documented procedures to ensure that medical devices returned to the organization are identified and distinguished from conforming product [see 6.4 d)]?
7.5.3.2 Traceability	
7.5.3.2.1 General	
	Has the organization established documented procedures for traceability?
	Do such procedures define the extent of product traceability and the records required (see 8.3 ,4.2.4 and 8.5)?
	Does the organization control and record the unique identification of the product, where traceability is a requirement (see 4.2.4)?

Doc. Reference	Adequate?	Stage I (clauses marked *)	Stage II

	REQUIREMENTS
EU	Does the manufacturer have procedures identifying the requirements of labeling and instructions for use as defined in MDD, Annex 1 point 13, and is regulations for CE marking included in these procedures. (MDD 3, Article 17 and Annex 12).
	Are language requirements defined in procedures for the information identified in MDD, Annex 1point 13 for the applicable markets.
7.5.3.2.2 Particular requirements for active implantable medical devices and	
	In defining the records required for traceability, does the organization include records of all components, materials and work environment conditions, if these could cause the medical device not to satisfy its specified requirements?
	Does the organization require that its agents or distributors maintain records of the distribution of medical devices to allow traceability and that such records be available for inspection?
	Are records of the name and address of the shipping package consignee maintained (see 4.2.4)?
7.5.3.3 Status identification	
	Does the organization identify the product status with respect to monitoring and measurement requirements?
	Is the identification of product status maintained throughout production, storage, installation and servicing of the product to ensure that only product that has passed the required inspections and tests (or released under an authorized concession) is dispatched, used or installed?
7.5.4 Customer property	
	Does the organization exercise care with customer property while it is under the organization's control or being used by the organization?

Doc. Reference	Adequate?	Stage I (clauses marked *)	Stage II
	.		

e medical devices

	REQUIREMENTS
	Does the organization identify, verify, protect and safeguard customer property provided for use or incorporation into the product?
	If any customer property is lost, damaged, or otherwise found to be unsuitable for use, is this reported to the customer and are records maintained (see 4.2.4)?
7.5.5 Preservation of product	
	Has the organization established documented procedures or documented work instructions for preserving the conformity of product during internal processing and delivery to the intended destination?
	Does this preservation include identification, handling, packaging, storage and protection, and also apply to the constituent parts of a product?
	Has the organization established documented procedures or documented work instructions for the control of product with a limited shelf-life or requiring special storage conditions?
	Are such special storage conditions controlled and recorded (see 4.2.4)?
7.6 Control of monitoring and measuring devices	
	Does the organization determine monitoring and measuring to be undertaken and the monitoring and measuring devices needed to provide evidence of conformity of product to determined requirements (guide reference 7.2.1)?
	Has the organization established documented procedures to ensure that monitoring and measurement can be carried out and are carried out in a manner that is consistent with the monitoring and measurement requirements?

Doc. Reference	Adequate?	Stage I (clauses marked *)	Stage II

	REQUIREMENTS
	Where necessary to ensure valid results, is measuring equipment:
	a) Calibrated or verified at specified intervals, or prior to use, against measurement standards traceable to international or national measurement standards; where no such standards exist, is the basis used for calibration or verification recorded?
	b) Adjusted or re-adjusted as necessary?
	c) Identified to enable the calibration status to be determined?
	d) Safeguarded from adjustments that would invalidate the measurement result?
	e) Protected from damage and deterioration during handling, maintenance and storage?
	Does the organization assess and record the validity of the previous measuring results when the equipment is found not to conform to requirements?
	Does the organization take appropriate action on the equipment and any product affected?
	Are records of the results of calibration and verification maintained (see 4.2.4)?
	When used in the monitoring and measurement of specified requirements, is the ability of computer software to satisfy the intended application confirmed prior to initial use and reconfirmed as necessary ?
8 Measurement, analysis and improvement	
8.1 General	

Doc. Reference	Adequate?	Stage I (clauses marked *)	Stage II

	REQUIREMENTS
	Does the organization plan and implement the monitoring, measurement, analysis and improvement processes needed:
	a) To demonstrate conformity of the product?
	b) To ensure conformity of the quality management system?
	c) To maintain the effectiveness of the quality management system?
	Does this include determination of applicable methods, including statistical techniques, and the extent of their use?
8.2 Monitoring and measurement	
8.2.1 Feedback	
	As one of the measurements of the performance of the quality management system, does the organization monitor information relating to whether the organization has met customer requirements?
	Have the methods for obtaining and using this information been determined?
	Has the organization established a documented procedure for a feedback system [see 7.2.3 c)] to provide early warning of quality problems and for input into the corrective and preventive action processes (see 8.5.2 and 8.5.3)?
	If national or regional regulations require the organization to gain experience from the post-production phase, does the review of this experience form part of the feedback system (see 8.5.1)?
Japan	Confirm that the personnel operating the Registered Manufacturing Site has determined and implemented effective arrangements for communicating with the Japanese Marketing Authorization Holder in relation to customer feedback, including customer complaints, and advisory notices [MHLW MO29 :169].
8.2.2 Internal audit	

Doc. Reference	Adequate?	Stage I (clauses marked *)	Stage II

	REQUIREMENTS
	Does the organization conduct internal audits at planned intervals to determine whether the quality management system
	a) Conforms to the planned arrangements (see 7.1), to the requirements of this International Standard and to the quality management system requirements established by the organization?
	b) Is effectively implemented and maintained?
	Is an audit programme planned, taking into consideration the status and importance of the processes and areas to be audited, as well as the results of previous audits?
	Are the audit criteria, scope, frequency and methods defined?
	Does selection of auditors and conduct of audits ensure objectivity and impartiality of the audit process (e.g. auditors shall not audit their own work)?
	Are the responsibilities and requirements for planning and conducting audits, and for reporting results and maintaining records (see 4.2.4) defined in a documented procedure?
	Does management responsible for the area being audited ensure that actions are taken without undue delay to eliminate detected nonconformities and their causes?
	Do follow-up activities include the verification of the actions taken and the reporting of verification results? (see 8.5.2)
8.2.3 Measurement and monitoring of processes	
	Does the organization apply suitable methods for monitoring and, where applicable, measurement of the quality management system processes?
	Do these methods demonstrate the ability of the processes to achieve planned results?

Doc. Reference	Adequate?	Stage I (clauses marked *)	Stage II

	REQUIREMENTS
	When planned results are not achieved, is correction and corrective action taken, as appropriate, to ensure conformity of the product?
8.2.4 Monitoring and measurement of product	
8.2.4.1 General requirements	
	Does the organization monitor and measure the characteristics of the product to verify that product requirements have been met?
	Is this carried out at appropriate stages of the product realization process in accordance with the planned arrangements (see 7.1) and documented procedures (see 7.5.1.1)?
	Is evidence of conformity with the acceptance criteria maintained?
	Do records indicate the person(s) authorizing release of the product (see 4.2.4)?
	Does the organization ensure that product release and service delivery do not proceed until the planned arrangements (see 7.1) have been satisfactorily completed?
8.2.4.2 Particular requirement for active implantable medical devices and ir	
	Does the organization record (see 4.2.4) the identity of personnel performing any inspection or testing?
8.3 Control of nonconforming product	
	Does the organization ensure that product which does not conform to product requirements is identified and controlled to prevent its unintended use or delivery?
	Are the controls and related responsibilities and authorities for dealing with nonconforming product defined in a documented procedure?

Doc. Reference	Adequate?	Stage I (clauses marked *)	Stage II
medical devices			

	REQUIREMENTS
	Does the organization deal with nonconforming product by one or more of the following ways?
	a) By taking action to eliminate the detected nonconformity
	b) By authorizing its use, release or acceptance under concession
	c) By taking action to preclude its original intended use or application
	Does the organization ensure that nonconforming product is accepted by concession only if regulatory requirements are met?
	Are records of the identity of the person(s) authorizing the concession maintained (see 4.2.4)?
	Are records of the nature of nonconformities and any subsequent actions taken, including concessions obtained maintained (see 4.2.4)?
	When nonconforming product is corrected, is it subject to re-verification to demonstrate conformity to the requirements?
	When nonconforming product is detected after delivery or use has started, does the organization take action appropriate to the effects, or potential effects, of the nonconformity?
	If product needs to be reworked (one or more times), does the organization document the rework process in a work instruction that has undergone the same authorization and approval procedure as the original work instruction?
	Prior to authorization and approval of the work instruction, is a determination of any adverse effect of the rework upon product made and documented (see 4.2.3 and 7.5.1)?
8.4 Analysis of data	

Doc. Reference	Adequate?	Stage I (clauses marked *)	Stage II

	REQUIREMENTS
	Does the organization establish documented procedures to determine, collect and analyse appropriate data to demonstrate the suitability and effectiveness of the quality management system and to evaluate if improvement of the effectiveness of the quality management system can be made?
	Does this include data generated as a result of monitoring and measurement and from other relevant sources?
	Does the analysis of data provide information relating to:
	a) Feedback (see 8.2.1)?
	b) Conformity to product requirements? (See 7.2.1)
	c) Characteristics and trends of processes and products including opportunities for preventive action?
	d) Suppliers?
	Are records of the results of the analysis of data maintained (see 4.2.4)?
8.5 Improvement	
8.5.1 General	
	Does the organization identify and implement any changes necessary to ensure and maintain the continued suitability and effectiveness of the quality management system through the use of the quality policy, quality objectives, audit results, analysis of data, corrective and preventive actions and management review?
	Does the organization establish documented procedures for the issue and implementation of advisory notices and are these procedures capable of being implemented at any time?

Doc. Reference	Adequate?	Stage I (clauses marked *)	Stage II

	REQUIREMENTS
Japan	Confirm that the personnel operating the Registered Manufacturing Site have determined and implemented effective arrangements for communicating with the Marketing Authorization Holder in relation to advisory notices [MHLW MO29 :169]. Note: Personnel operating Registered Manufacturing Sites are not required to report any advisory notice directly to the regulatory authority but shall communicate with the Marketing Authorization Holder, so the MAH can take any necessary regulatory actions.
EU	Are the procedures for Vigilance reporting in conformance with MDD Annex II, V, and VI (MEDDEV 1-2.12)
	Are records of all customer complaint investigations maintained (see 4.2.4)?
	If investigation determines that the activities outside the organization contributed to the customer complaint, is relevant information exchanged between the organizations involved (see 4.1)?
	If any customer complaint is not followed by corrective and/or preventive action, is the reason authorized (see 5.5.1) and recorded (see 4.2.4)?
	If national or regional regulations require notification of adverse events that meet specific reporting criteria, does the organization establish documented procedures to such notification to regulatory authorities?
Japan	Verify that the person operating the Registered Manufacturing Site provides events which meet the criteria defined by the Ordinance for Enforcement of PMD Act Article 2) 20-228) to the MarketingAuthorization Holder in a timely manner.

Doc. Reference	Adequate?	Stage I (clauses marked *)	Stage II

	REQUIREMENTS
EU	Are procedures for the reporting of recall to the relevant competent authority and the NB compliant? (MDD, Annex II, V, VI, 3.1)
8.5.2 Corrective action	
	Does the organization take action to eliminate the cause of nonconformities in order to prevent recurrence and are corrective actions appropriate to the effects of the nonconformities encountered?
	Has a documented procedure been established to define requirements for:
	a) Reviewing nonconformities (including customer complaints)?
	b) Determining the causes of nonconformities?
	c) Evaluating the need for action to ensure that nonconformities do no recur?
	d) Determining and implementing action needed, including, if appropriate, updating documentation (see 4.2)?
	e) Recording of the results of any investigation and of action taken (see 4.2.4)?
	f) Reviewing the corrective action taken and its effectiveness?
8.5.3 Preventive action	
	Does the organization determine action to eliminate the causes of potential nonconformities in order to prevent their occurrence and are preventive actions appropriate to the effects of the potential problems?

Doc. Reference	Adequate?	Stage I (clauses marked *)	Stage II

	REQUIREMENTS
	Has a documented procedure been established to define requirements for:
	a) Determining potential nonconformities and their causes?
	b) Evaluating the need for action to prevent occurrence of nonconformities?
	c) Determining and implementing action needed?
	d) Recording of the results of any investigations and of action taken (see 4.2.4)?
	e) Reviewing preventive action taken and its effectiveness?

Doc. Reference	Adequate?	Stage I (clauses marked *)	Stage II

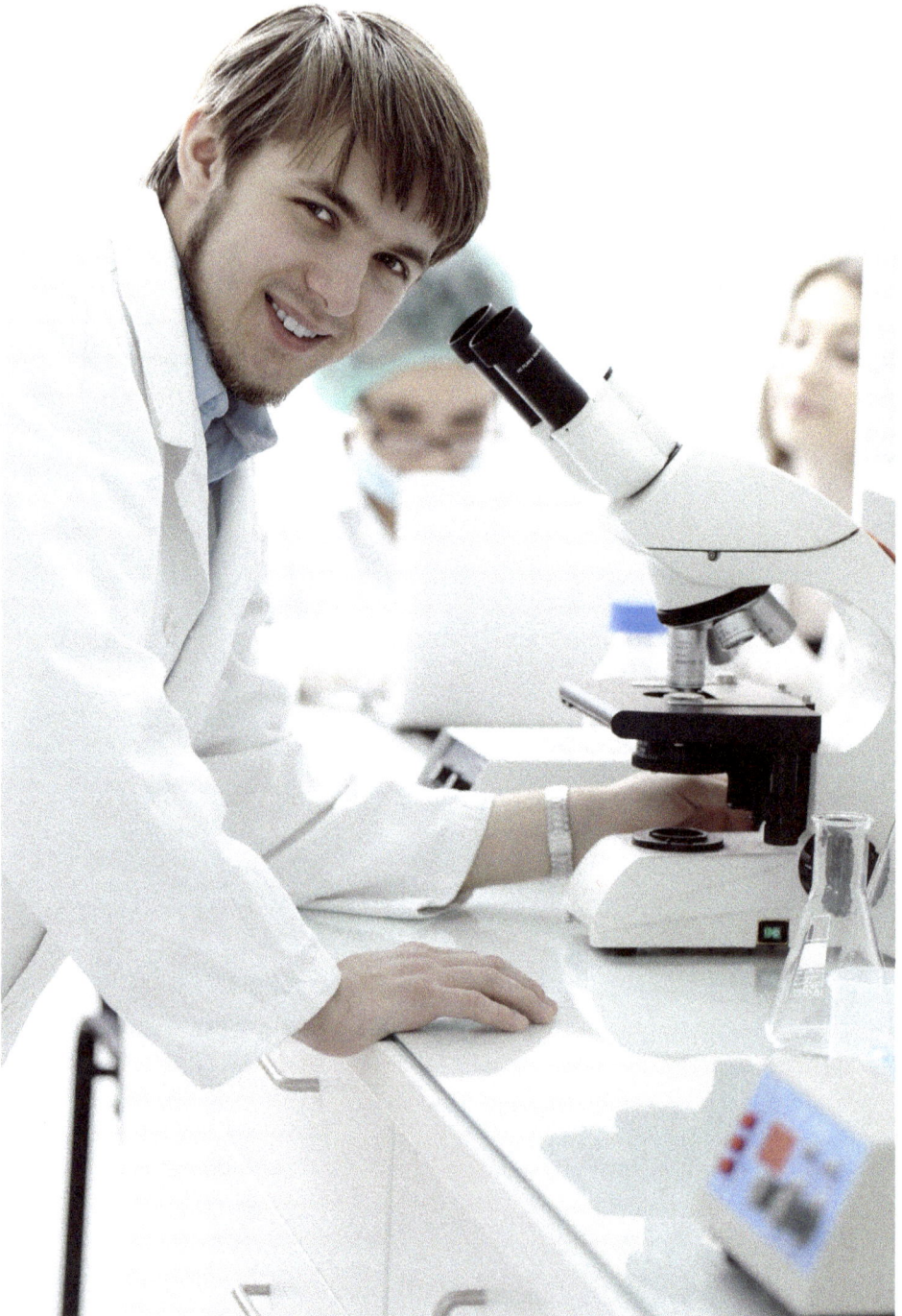

MDSAP
ISO 13485 Requirements &

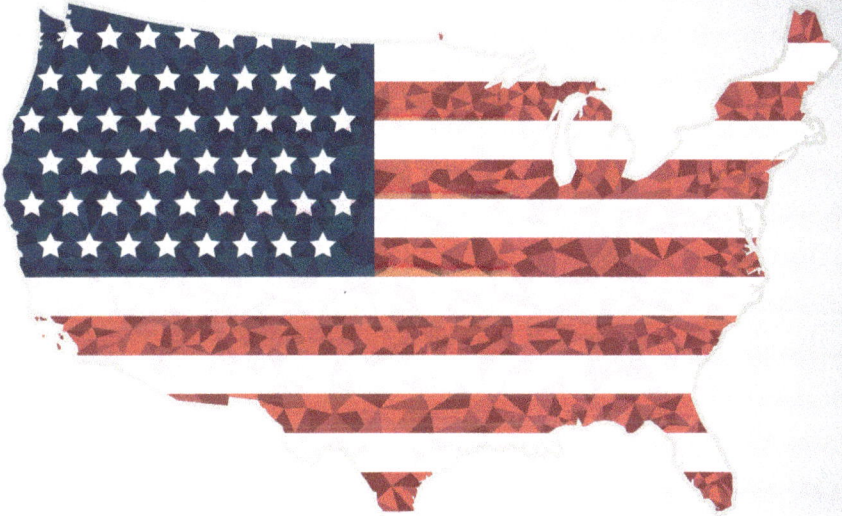

Management

The intent of the Management Process is to provide adequate resources for device design, manufacturing, quality assurance, distribution, installation, and servicing activities; to assure the quality management system is functioning properly and effectively; and to monitor the quality management system and make necessary adjustments. A quality management system that has been implemented effectively and is monitored to identify and address existing and potential problems is more likely to produce medical devices that function as intended.

The management representative is responsible for ensuring that the requirements of the quality management system have been effectively defined, documented, implemented, and maintained. Prior to the audit of a process, it may be helpful to interview the management representative (or designee) to obtain an overview of the process and a feel for management's knowledge and understanding of the process.

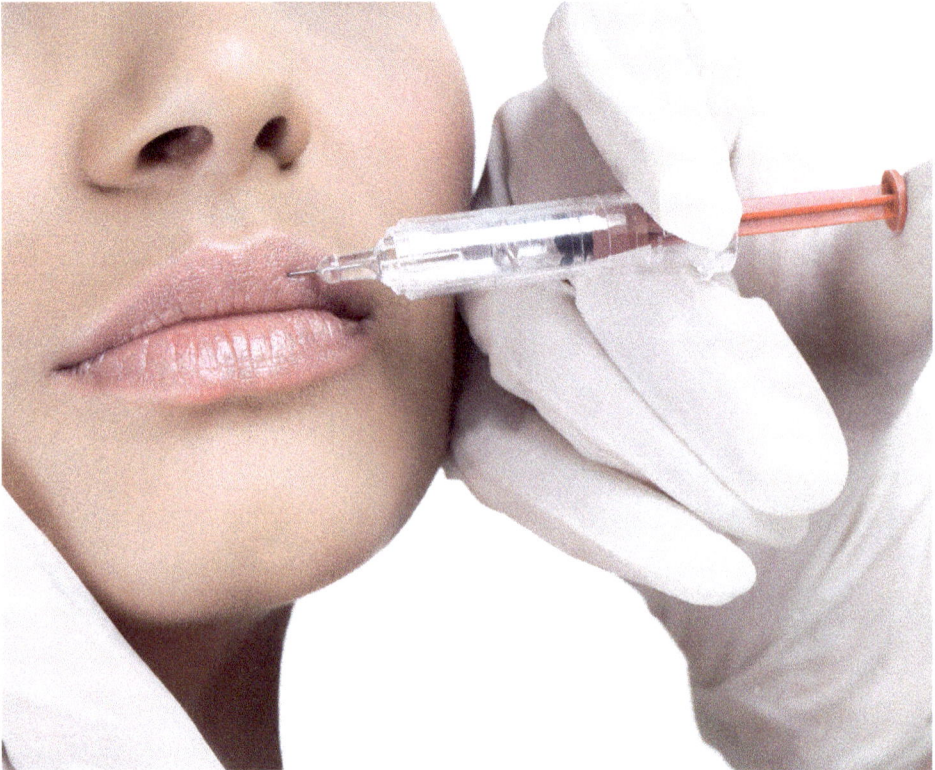

Clause and Regulation:
ISO 13485:2016: 4.1.1, 4.1.2, 4.1.3, 4.2.2, 4.1.4, 5.4.2;
FDA: 21 CFR 820.20, FDA: 21 CFR 820.20(b),
FDA: 21CFR 820.20(a), FDA: 21 CFR 820.40, 820.180
FDA: 21 CFR 820.20(a), 820.5,

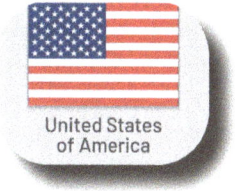

United States
of America

Verify that electronic records and documents have backups
[21 CFR 820.180].
Confirm that the medical device organization has defined, documented, and implemented procedures for control of quality management system documents and records. Evidence that these controls are effective can be ascertained through the audit of the other quality management system processes. For example, evidence that the document controls process is ineffective might be the observation of obsolete procedures being used or required records being unavailable.
Ensure at least one copy of obsolete controlled documents is maintained. Confirm that top management has shown commitment to the risk management process by ensuring the provision of adequate resources and the assignment of qualified personnel for risk management activities. Risk-based decisions occur throughout the various quality management system processes. Top management is responsible for defining and documenting the policy for determining criteria for risk acceptability. Additionally, ensure top management reviews the suitability of the risk management process. This review may be part of the management review. Previously unidentified risks discovered during production and post-production of the medical device may indicate a need to improve the risk management process. Each medical device organization must decide how much risk is acceptable.

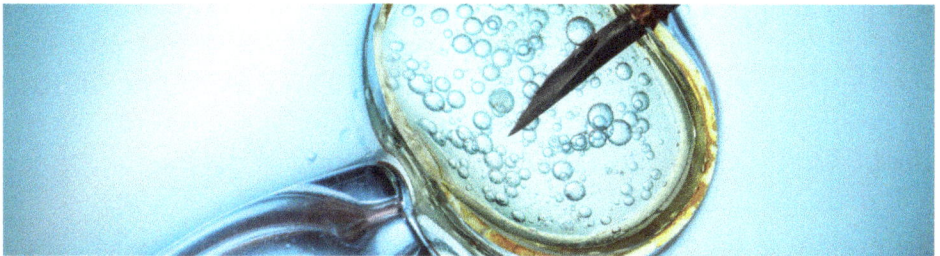

Device Marketing Authorization and Facility Registration

The Device Marketing Authorization and Facility Registration process may be audited as a linkage from the Management process and/or the Design and Development process.

ISO: ISO 13485:2016: 4.1.1, 4.2.1, 5.2, 7.2.1, 7.2.3

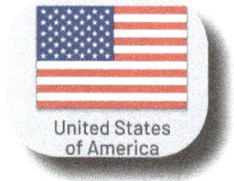

United States
of America

21 CFR 807 - Establishment Registration and Device Listing for Manufacturers and Initial Importers of Devices.

Establishment means a place of business under one management at one general physical location at which a device is manufactured, assembled, or otherwise processed.

Owner or operator means the corporation, subsidiary, affiliated company, partnership, or proprietor directly responsible for the activities of the registering establishment.

Owner or operator must register the establishment and submit listing information to Food and Drug Administration (FDA) for those devices in commercial distribution, regardless of classification.

The registration and listing requirements must pertain to any person who:

- Initiates or develops specifications for a device that is to be manufactured by a second party for commercial distribution by the person initiating specifications

- Manufactures for commercial distribution a device either for itself or for another person; regardless of whether the manufacturer places the device into commercial distribution or returns the device to the customer

- Repackages or relabels a device

-Acts as an initial importer, except that initial importers may fulfill their listing obligation for any device for which they did not initiate or develop the specifications for the device or repackage or relabel the device by submitting the name and address of the manufacturer

- Manufactures components or accessories which are ready to be used for any intended health-related purpose and are packaged or

labeled for commercial distribution for such purpose
- Sterilizes or otherwise makes a device for or on behalf of a specification developer or any other person
- Acts as a complaint file establishment
- Is a device establishment located in a foreign trade zone.
21 CFR 807.81- Premarket Notification:
Each person who is required to register his establishment pursuant to 807.20 must submit a premarket notification submission to the Food and Drug Administration at least 90 days before he proposes to begin the introduction or delivery for introduction into interstate commerce for commercial distribution of a device intended for human use which meets any of the following criteria:
- The device is being introduced into commercial distribution for the first time; that is, the device is not of the same type as, or is not substantially equivalent to, (i) a device in commercial distribution before May 28, 1976, or (ii) a device introduced for commercial distribution after May 28, 1976, that has subsequently been reclassified into class I or II.
- The device is being introduced into commercial distribution for the first time by a person required to register.
21 CFR 814 – Premarket Approval
A Premarket approval is required for any FDA class III device that was not on the market (introduced or delivered for introduction into commerce for commercial distribution) before May 28, 1976, and is not substantially equivalent to a device on the market before May 28, 1976, or to a device first marketed on, or after that date, which has been classified into class I or class II.
21 CFR 807 - Establishment Registration and Device Listing for Manufacturers and Initial Importers of Devices.
Update the device listing information during each June and December or, at its discretion, at the time the change occurs. Conditions that require updating and information to be submitted for each of these updates are as follows:
- If an owner or operator introduces into commercial distribution a device identified with a classification name not currently listed by the owner or operator
- If an owner or operator discontinues commercial distribution of all

devices in the same device class

Update registration if changes in individual ownership, corporate or partnership structure, or location of at the time of annual registration, or by letter if the changes occur at other times. This information must be submitted within 30 days of such changes. Changes in the names of officers and/or directors of the corporation(s) must be filed with the establishment's official correspondent and must be provided to the Food and Drug Administration upon receipt of a written request for this information.

21 CFR 807.81- Premarket Notification:

A new complete 510(k) application is required for changes or modifications to an existing device, where the modifications could significantly affect the safety or effectiveness of the device, or the device is to be marketed for a new or different indication. All changes in indications for use require the submission of a 510(k).

Examples of modifications that may require a 510(k) submission include, but are not limited to, the following:
- Sterilization method
- Structural material
- Manufacturing method
- Operating parameters or conditions for use
- Patient or user safety features
- Sterile barrier packaging material
- Stability or expiration claims
- Design.

21 CFR 814.39 – PMA Supplements

After FDA's approval of a PMA, an applicant shall submit a PMA supplement for review and approval by FDA before making a change affecting the safety or effectiveness of the device for which the applicant has an approved PMA. While the burden for determining whether a supplement is required is primarily on the PMA holder, changes for which an applicant shall submit a PMA supplement include, but are not limited to, the following types of changes if they affect the safety or effectiveness of the device:
- New indications for use of the device
- Labeling changes
- The use of a different facility or establishment to manufacture,

process, or package the device
- Changes in sterilization procedures
- Changes in packaging
- Changes in the performance or design specifications, circuits, components, ingredients, principle of operation, or physical layout of the device
- Extension of the expiration date of the device based on data obtained under a new or revised stability or sterility testing protocol that has not been approved by FDA
- An applicant may make a change in a device after FDA's approval of a PMA for the device without submitting a PMA supplement if the change does not affect the device's safety or effectiveness and the change is reported to FDA in post approval periodic reports required as a condition to approval of the device, e.g., an editorial change in labeling which does not affect the safety or effectiveness of the device.

Clause and Regulation
ISO: ISO 13485:2016: 4.2.1, 8.1, 8.2.1, 8.2.6, 8.5
FDA: 21 CFR 820.100(a), 21 CFR 820.100 (a)(2)

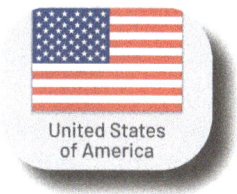

United States
of America

Measurement, Analysis and Improvement

One of the most important activities in the quality management system is the identification of existing and potential causes of product and quality problems. Such causes must be identified so that appropriate and effective corrective or preventive actions can take place. These activities are carried out under the Measurement, Analysis and Improvement process.

Verify procedures ensure that information related to quality problems or nonconforming product is disseminated to those directly responsible for assuring the quality of such product or the prevention of problems [21 CFR 820.100(a)(6)].

Confirm procedures provide for the submission of relevant information on identified quality problems, as well as corrective and preventive actions, for management review
[21 CFR 820.100(a)(7)].

Medical Device Adverse Events and Advisory Notices Reporting
The Medical Device Adverse Events and Advisory Notices Reporting
process may be audited as a linkage from the Measurement, Analysis
and Improvement process.

Clause and Regulation
ISO: ISO 13485:2016: 4.2.1, 7.2.3, 8.2.2, 8.2.2, 8.2.3,
8.3.3

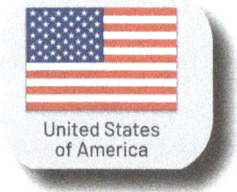

United States
of America

21 CFR 803: Medical Device Reporting
Determine whether the manufacturer has developed a process for
reporting to FDA incidents involving device-related deaths, serious
injuries, and reportable malfunctions that occur within and outside
the United States if the same or similar device is marketed to the
United States.
Confirm that the manufacturer has developed, maintained, and im-
plemented written medical device reporting (MDR) procedures for
the following:
- Internal processes that provide for:
- Timely and effective identification, communication, and evaluation
of events that may be subject to MDR requirements
- A standardized review process or procedure for determining when
an event meets the criteria for reporting
- Timely transmission of complete medical device reports to FDA
- Documentation and recordkeeping requirements for:
- Information that was evaluated to determine if an event was report-
able;
- All medical device reports and information submitted to FDA
- Processes that ensure access to information that facilitates timely
follow-up and audit.
Verify that reports are made within 30 calendar days after the day
that the manufacturer receives or otherwise becomes aware of infor-
mation, from any source, that reasonably suggests that a device that
is marketed may have caused or contributed to a death or serious
injury:
- Confirm the manufacturer's MDR files contain the following:
- Information (or references to information) related to the ad-

verse event, including all documentation of deliberations and decision-making processes used to determine if a device- related death, serious injury, or malfunction was or was not reportable to FDA

- Copies of all MDR forms and other information related to the event submitted to FDA.

If a device has malfunctioned and this device or a similar device that is marketed would be likely to cause or contribute to a death or serious injury, if the malfunction were to recur, quarterly summary reporting is acceptable for most device product codes.

If the manufacturer maintains MDR event files as part of the complaint file, ensure that the manufacturer has prominently identified these records as MDR reportable events. FDA will not consider a submitted MDR report to comply with 21 CFR 803 unless the manufacturer evaluates an event in accordance with the quality management system requirements. Confirm that the manufacturer has documented and maintained in the MDR event files an explanation of why the manufacturer did not submit or could not obtain any information required by 21 CFR 803, as well as the results of the evaluation of each event.

Compare the information submitted on the individual medical device report to the information contained in the associated complaint and confirm the medical device report contains all information related to the event that is reasonably known to the manufacturer.

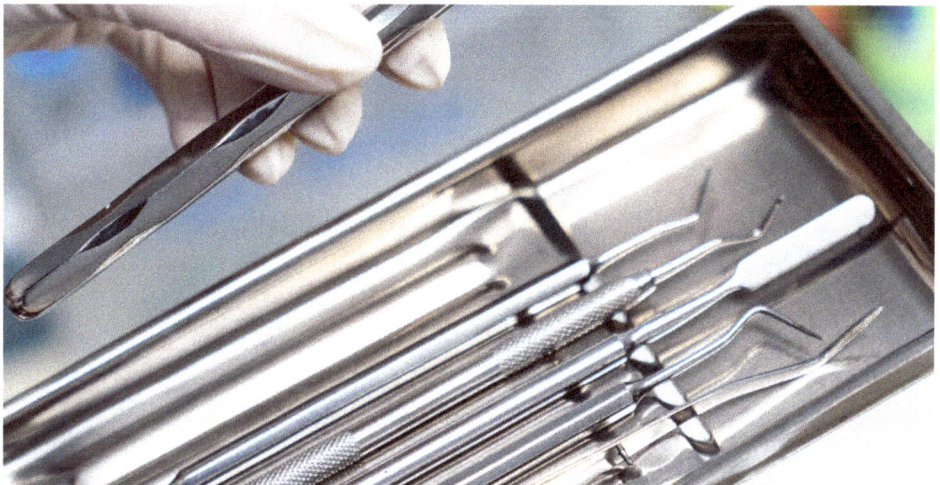

Design and Development

The purpose of the Design and Development process is to control the design of a medical device and to assure that the device meets user needs, intended use, and its specified requirements. Attention to design and development planning, identifying design inputs, developing design outputs, verifying that design outputs meet design inputs, validating the design, controlling design changes, reviewing design results, transferring the design to production, and compiling the appropriate records will help a medical device organization assure that resulting designs will meet user needs, intended uses, and requirements. Review of the Design and Development process will also provide an opportunity to evaluate how the medical device organization has utilized risk management activities to ensure design inputs are comprehensive and meet user needs, to confirm that risk control measures that were planned have been implemented in the design, and to verify that risk control measures are effective in controlling or reducing risk.

Clause and Regulation
ISO: ISO 13485:2016: 4.1.1, 4.2.1, 7.1, 7.3.10, 7.3.2
FDA: 21 CFR 820.30(a), 820.30(b), 820.30(j)

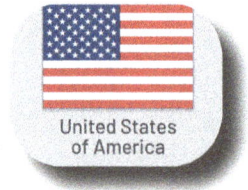

United States
of America

Verify that the design input procedures contain a mechanism for addressing incomplete, ambiguous, or conflicting requirements [21 CFR 820.30(c)].

Confirm that the manufacturer has identified the possible hazards associated with the device in both normal and fault conditions. The risks associated with the hazards, including those resulting from user error, should be calculated in both normal and fault conditions.
If any risk is judged to be unacceptable, it should be reduced to acceptable levels by the appropriate means. Ensure changes to the device to eliminate or minimize hazards do not introduce new hazards [21 CFR 820.30(g); preamble comment 83].

Production and Service Controls

The purpose of the Production and Service Controls process is to manufacture products that meet specifications. Developing processes that are adequate to produce devices that meet specifications, validating (or fully verifying the results of) those processes, and monitoring and controlling those processes are all steps that help assure the result will be devices that meet specified requirements. After completing the audit of the medical device organization's Production and Service Controls process, the audit team will return to the Management process to make a final decision of whether top management ensures that an adequate and effective quality management system has been established and maintained at the medical device organization.

Clause and Regulation
ISO: ISO 13485:2016: 7.1, 7.2.1, 7.5.1, 8.2.5, 8.2.6
FDA: 21 CFR 801, 820.30(b), 820.20(a), 820.30(h), 820.70(a), 830

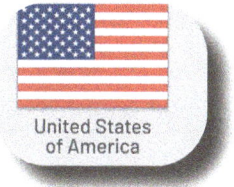

United States
of America

Confirm that the medical device organization has determined the applicability of unique device identifier requirements per 21 CFR 801 and 21 CFR 830, has obtained the unique device identifiers from an FDA-accredited UDI-issuing agency, and the required data elements have been entered in the Global Unique Device Identification Database (GUDID) [21 CFR 801, 830].

Process validation is required for sterilization, aseptic processing, injection molding, and welding [21 CFR 820.75; preamble comment 143].

If a control number is required for traceability, confirm that a control number is on, or accompanies the device throughout distribution [21 CFR 820.120(e)].

Confirm that labeling is stored in a manner that provides proper identification and prevents mix-ups. Verify labeling and packaging operations are controlled to prevent labeling mix-ups [21 CFR 820.120(c) and (d)].

Verify that the label and labeling used for each production unit, lot, or batch are documented in the batch record, as well as any control numbers used [21 CFR 820.120(e), 820.184(e)].

Reviewing a validation

During review of a validation study, determine when applicable whether:

- The instruments used to generate the data were properly calibrated and maintained
- Predetermined product and process specifications were established
- Sampling plans used to collect test samples are based on a statistically valid rationale
- Data demonstrates predetermined specifications were met consistently
- Process tolerance limits were challenged
- Process equipment was properly installed, adjusted, and maintained
- Process monitoring instruments were properly calibrated and maintained
- Changes to the validated process were appropriately challenged (if applicable)
- Process operators were appropriately qualified.

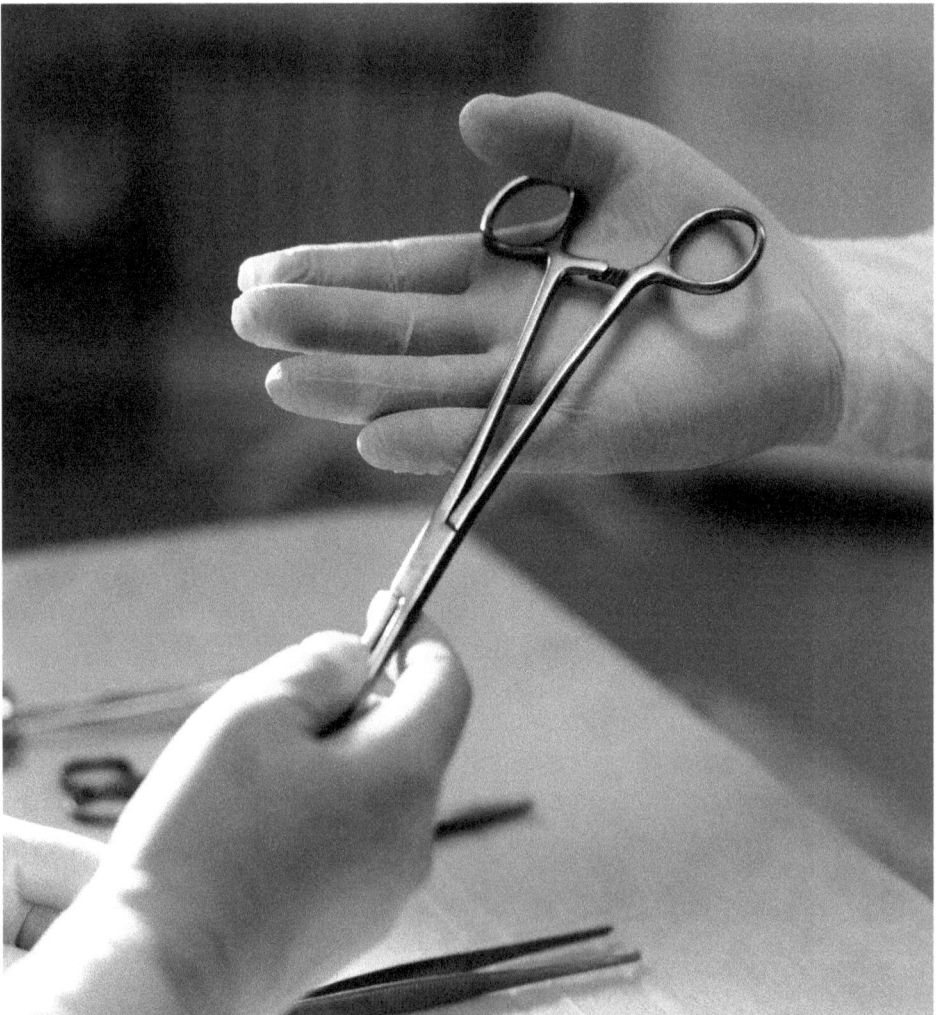

Purchasing

The intent of the Purchasing process is to ensure that purchased, sub-contracted, or otherwise received products and services conform to specified requirements. The medical device organization is expected to establish and maintain documented controls for planning and performing purchasing activities. The controls necessary depend on the effect of the product on the quality, safety, and effectiveness of the finished device. Effective purchasing processes incorporate purchasing requirements and specifications, the selection of acceptable suppliers based on the capability of the suppliers to provide acceptable product, the performance of necessary acceptance activities, and maintenance of the required quality records.

The management representative is responsible for ensuring that the requirements of the quality management system have been effectively defined, documented, implemented, and maintained. Prior to the audit of a process, it may be helpful to interview the management representative to obtain an overview of the process and a feel for management's knowledge and understanding of the process.

Clause and Regulation
ISO: ISO: ISO 13485:2016: 4.1.2, 4.1.3, 4.1.5, 7.1, 7.4.1, 7.4.2, 7.4.3

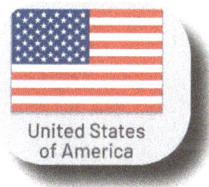

United States
of America

Planning

In planning product realization, the medical device organization must determine as appropriate the quality objectives and requirements for the purchased products, the processes, documents, and resources specific to the purchased products, the criteria for purchased product acceptance, and the required verification, monitoring, inspection, and test activities specific to the purchased products. Planning of product realization often begins in the design and development of the product, including the translation of the design into production specifications. The translation of the design into production specifications includes the establishment of specified requirements for purchased product.

Quality objectives

Quality objectives are typically expressed as a measurable target or goal. The planning of product realization should include consideration of how the purchased product, the criteria for purchased product acceptance, and the required verification, monitoring, inspection, and test activities specific to the purchased product will achieve the quality objectives.

- Some examples of QOB include:
- Number of complaints -v- number of parts shipped
- On-time delivery %
- Supplier parts rejected
- Comparison of internal audit findings -v- external audit findings
- Achieving a certain accuracy if you're developing product - based software
- Annual Post-market surveillance
- Auditing our system for regulatory compliance

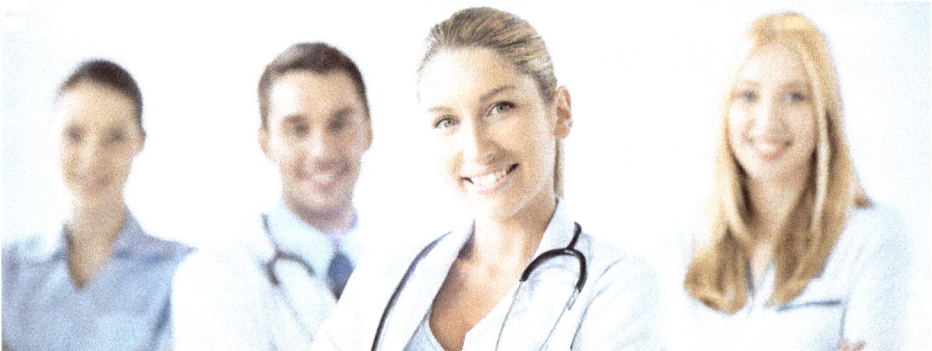

Some managers believe that the reward for hard work should be a paycheck. That's sort of like telling your children that they get to eat for doing something you're proud of. Employees are not children, but you are responsible for developing them into more valuable employees so that they can be promoted. If there is no incentive, your team will not be engaged. Therefore, pick a reward that is proportional to the bottom-line impact. Five percent of the bottom-line impact is what I like to target, but you would be amazed at how effective a few small rewards at each milestone can be. If you have trouble getting management approval for rewards, remind your boss of the bottom-line impact and link the rewards closely to the impact.

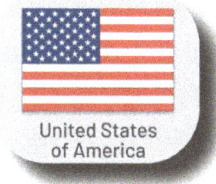

MDSAP
Audit Checklist

	REQUIREMENTS

4 Quality management system	
4.1 General requirements	
	Has the organization:
	a) identified the processes needed for the quality management system and their application throughout the organization (see 1.2)?
	b) determined the sequence and interaction of these processes?
	c) determined criteria and methods needed to ensure that both the operation and control of these processes are effective?
	d) ensured the availability of resources and information necessary to support the operation and monitoring of their processes?
	e) monitored, measured, and analyzed these processes
	f) implemented actions necessary to achieve planned results and maintain the effectiveness of these processes?
	Does the organization manage these processes in accordance with the requirements of this International Standard?
	Where an organization chooses to outsource any process that affects product conformity with requirements, does the organization ensure control over such processes?
	Is the control of such outsourced processes identified within the quality management system? (see 8.5.1)
4.2.1 General	

Doc. Reference	Adequate?	Stage I (clauses marked *)	Stage II
	Y/N	Initial›s	Initial›s

	REQUIREMENTS
	Does the quality management system documentation include:
	a) documented statements of a quality policy and quality objectives?
	b) a quality manual?
	c) documented procedures required by this international standard?
	d) documents needed by the organization to ensure the effective planning, operation and control of its processes?
	e) records required by this International Standard (see 4.2.4)?
	f) any other documentation specified by national or regional regulations?
	Has the organization established and maintained a file for each type or model of medical device either containing or identifying documents defining product specifications and quality system requirements (see 4.2.3)?
	Do these documents define the complete manufacturing process and, if applicable, installation and servicing?
Canada	Verify that the manufacturer maintains distribution records that contain sufficient information to permit complete and rapid withdrawal of the medical device from the market [CMDR 53-52].
	Verify that distribution records of a device are retained by the manufacturer in a manner that will allow for timely retrieval, for the longer of (a) the projected useful life of the device; and (b) two years after the date the device was shipped [CMDR 56-55].

Doc. Reference	Adequate?	Stage I (clauses marked *)	Stage II

	REQUIREMENTS
US	Verify that the manufacturer maintains distribution records which include or refer to the location of the name and address of the initial consignee, the identification and quantity of devices shipped; and any control numbers used [21 CFR 820.160(b)].
EU	Does the file contain or refer to the location of objective evidence establishing the safety and effectiveness of the device as required by Annex 1 of the MDD? (MDD Annex I)
4.2.2 Quality manual	
	Has the organization established and maintained a quality manual that includes:
	a) the scope of the quality management system, including details of and justification for any exclusion and/or non-application (see 1.2)?
	b) the documented procedures established for the quality management system, or reference to them?
	c) a description of the interaction between the processes of the quality management system?
	Does the quality manual outline the structure of the documentation used in the quality management system?
US	Confirm the establishment is registered with FDA and devices marketed to the United States are listed. Confirm the manufacturer has submitted a pre-market notification or approval (as applicable) to FDA prior to marketing the device in the United States [21 CFR 807].
EU	Are the applicable sections of the Medical Device Directive (MDD) included in the specified requirements throughout the documented quality system? Interpretation: A statement only indicating compliance/conformity with the relevant international or EU regulatory requirements is not acceptable.
4.2.3 Control of documents	

Doc. Reference	Adequate?	Stage I (clauses marked *)	Stage II

	REQUIREMENTS
	Are documents required by the quality management system controlled?
	Is a documented procedure established to define the controls needed:
	a) To review and approve documents for adequacy prior to issue?
	b) To review and update as necessary and re-approve documents?
	c) To ensure that changes and the current revision status of documents are identified?
	d) To ensure that relevant versions of applicable documents are available at points of use?
	e) To ensure the documents remain legible and readily identifiable?
	f) To ensure that documents of external origin are identified and their distribution controlled?
	g) To prevent the unintended use of obsolete documents and to apply suitable identification to them if they are retained for any purpose?
	Does the organization ensure that changes to documents are reviewed and approved either by the original approving function or another designated function which has access to pertinent background information upon which to base its decisions?
	Does the organization define the period for which at least one copy of obsolete controlled documents shall be retained?
	Does this period ensure that documents to which medical devices have been manufactured and tested are available for at least the lifetime of the medical device as defined by the organization, but not less than the retention period of any resulting record (see 4.2.4), or as specified by relevant regulatory requirements?

Doc. Reference	Adequate?	Stage I (clauses marked *)	Stage II

	REQUIREMENTS
US	Confirm that approved changes to documents are communicated to the appropriate personnel in a timely manner [21 CFR 820.40(b)].
4.2.4 Control of quality records	
	Are records established and maintained to provide evidence of conformity to requirements and of the effective operation of the quality management system?
	Do records remain legible, readily identifiable and retrievable?
	Has a documented procedure been established to define the controls needed for the identification, storage, protection, retrieval, retention time and disposition of records?
	Does the organization retain the records for a period of time at least equivalent to the lifetime of the medical device as defined by the organization, but not less than two years from the date of product release by the organization or as specified by relevant regulatory requirements?
EU	Has the manufacturer retained for a period ending at least five years after the last product has been manufactured, the records listed in Annex II, 6.1 or Annex V, 5.1 or Annex VI, 5.1 (whichever applies)
5 Management responsibility	
5.1 Management commitment	

Doc. Reference	Adequate?	Stage I (clauses marked *)	Stage II

	REQUIREMENTS
	Has top management provided evidence of its commitment to the development and implementation of the quality management system and maintaining its effectiveness by:
	a) Communicating to the organization the importance of meeting customer as well as statutory and regulatory requirements?
	b) Establishing the quality policy?
	c) Ensuring that quality objectives are established?
	d) Conducting management reviews?
	e) Ensuring the availability of resources?
5.2 Customer focus	
	Does top management ensure that customer requirements are determined and met (see 7.2.1 and 8.2.1)?
5.3 Quality policy	
	Does top management ensure that the quality policy
	a) Is appropriate to the purpose of the organization?
	b) Includes a commitment to comply with requirements and to maintain the effectiveness of the quality management system?
	c) Provides a framework for establishing and reviewing quality objectives?
	d) Is communicated and understood within the organization?
	e) Is reviewed for continuing suitability?
5.4 Planning	
5.4.1 Quality objectives	
	Does top management ensure that quality objectives, including those needed to meet requirements for product (see 7.1a), are established at relevant functions and levels within the organization?
	Are quality objectives measurable?

Doc. Reference	Adequate?	Stage I (clauses marked *)	Stage II

	REQUIREMENTS	
	Are quality objectives consistent with the quality policy?	
5.4.2 Quality management system planning		
	Has top management ensured that:	
	a) The planning of the quality management system is carried out in order to meet the requirements given in 4.1, as well as the quality objectives?	
	b) The integrity of the quality management system is maintained when changes to the quality management system are planned and implemented?	
US	Confirm the organization has established a quality plan which defines the quality practices, resources, and activities relevant to devices that are designed and manufactured (21 CFR 820.20(d))	
5.5 Responsibility, authority and communication		
5.5.1 Responsibility and authority		
	Has top management ensured that responsibilities and authorities were defined, documented and communicated within the organization?	
	Has top management established the interrelation of all personnel who manage, perform and verify work affecting quality, and ensured the independence and authority necessary to perform these tasks?	
5.5.2 Management representative		

Doc. Reference	Adequate?	Stage I (clauses marked *)	Stage II

	REQUIREMENTS
	Has top management appointed a member of management who, irrespective of other responsibilities, has responsibility and authority that includes:
	a) Ensuring that processes needed for the quality management system are established, implemented, and maintained?
	b) Reporting to top management on the performance of the quality management system and any need for improvement (see 8.5)?
	c) Ensuring the promotion of awareness of regulatory and customer requirements throughout the organization?
5.5.3 Internal communication	
	Has top management ensured that appropriate communication processes have been established within the organization and that communication takes place regarding the effectiveness of the quality management system?
5.6 Management review	
5.6.1 General	
	Does top management review the organization's quality management system, at planned intervals, to ensure its continuing suitability, adequacy and effectiveness?
	Does this review include assessing opportunities for improvement and the need for changes to the quality management system, including the quality policy and quality objectives?
	Are records from management reviews maintained (see 4.2.4)?
5.6.2 Review input	

Doc. Reference	Adequate?	Stage I (clauses marked *)	Stage II

	REQUIREMENTS
	Does the input to management review include information on:
	a) Results of audits?
	b) Customer feedback?
	c) Process performance and product conformity?
	d) Status of preventive and corrective actions?
	e) Follow-up actions from previous management reviews?
	f) Changes that could affect the quality management system?
	g) Recommendations for improvement?
	h) New or revised regulatory requirements?
5.6.3 Review output	
	Does output from the management review include any decisions and actions related to:
	a) Improvements needed to maintain the effectiveness of the quality management system and its processes?
	b) Improvement of product related to customer requirements?
	c) Resource needs?
6 Resource management	
6.1 Provision of resources	
	Does the organization determine and provide the resources needed:
	a) To implement the quality management system and to maintain its effectiveness?
	b) To meet regulatory and customer requirements?
6.2 Human resources	
6.2.1 General	
	Are personnel performing work affecting product quality competent on the basis of appropriate education, training, skills and experience?
6.2.2 Competence, awareness and training	

Doc. Reference	Adequate?	Stage I (clauses marked *)	Stage II

	REQUIREMENTS
	Does the organization:
	a) determine the necessary competence for personnel performing work affecting product quality?
	b) Provide training or take other actions to satisfy these needs?
	c) Evaluate the effectiveness of actions taken?
	d) Ensure that its personnel are aware of the relevance and importance of their activities and how they contribute to the achievement of the quality objectives?
	e) Maintain appropriate records of education, training, skills and experience (see 4.2.4)?
US	Verify that resources include the assignment of trained personnel to meet the requirements of 21 CFR Part 820, including management, performance of work, assessment activities, and internal quality audits [21 CFR 820.20(b)(2)].
6.3 Infrastructure	
	Does the organization determine, provide and maintain the infrastructure needed to achieve conformity to product requirements?
	Infrastructure includes, as applicable:
	a) Buildings, workspace and associated utilities
	b) Process equipment, both hardware and software
	c) Supporting services such as transport or communication
	Does the organization establish documented requirements for maintenance activities, including their frequency, when such activities or lack thereof can affect product quality?
	Are records of such maintenance maintained (see 4.2.4)?
	Has the organization determined and does it manage the work environment needed to achieve conformity to product requirements?

Doc. Reference	Adequate?	Stage I (clauses marked *)	Stage II

	REQUIREMENTS
	a) Has the organization established documented requirements for health, cleanliness and clothing of personnel if contact between such personnel and the product or work environment could adversely affect the quality of the product (see 7.5.1.2.1)?
	b) If work environment conditions can have an adverse effect on product quality, has organization established documented requirements for the work environment conditions and documented procedures or work instructions to monitor and control these work environment conditions (see 7.5.1.2.1)?
	c) Does the organization ensure that all personnel who are required to work temporarily under special environmental conditions within the work environment are appropriately trained or supervised by a trained person [see 6.2.2 b)]?
	d) If appropriate, are special arrangements established and documented for the control of contaminated or potentially contaminated product in order to prevent contamination of other product, the work environment or personnel (see 7.5.3.1)?
7 Product realization	
7.1 Planning of product realization	
	Has the organization planned and developed the processes needed for product realization?
	Is the planning of product realization consistent with the requirements of the other processes of the quality management system (see 4.1)?

Doc. Reference	Adequate?	Stage I (clauses marked *)	Stage II

	REQUIREMENTS
	In planning product realization, has the organization determined the following, as appropriate:
	a) Quality objectives and requirements for products?
	b) The need to establish processes, documents, and provide resources specific to the product?
	c) Required verification, validation, monitoring, inspection and test activities specific to the product and the criteria for product acceptance?
	d) Records needed to provide evidence that the realization processes and resulting product meet requirements (see 4.2.4)?
	Is the output of this planning in a form suitable for the organization's method of operations?
	Does the organization establish documented requirements for risk management throughout product realization and are records arising from risk management maintained (see 4.2.4)?
US	Confirm that the manufacturer has identified the possible hazards associated with the device in both normal and fault conditions. The risks associated with the hazards, including those resulting from user error, should be calculated in both normal and fault conditions. If any risk is judged to be unacceptable, it should be reduced to acceptable levels by the appropriate means. Ensure changes to the device to eliminate or minimize hazards do not introduce new hazards [21 CFR 820.30(g); preamble comment 83].
EU	Does the supplier evaluate the need for risk analysis throughout the design process and maintain records of any risk analysis performed? (MDD Annex 1)
	7.2.1 Determination of requirements related to the product

Doc. Reference	Adequate?	Stage I (clauses marked *)	Stage II

	REQUIREMENTS
	Has the organization determined:
	a) Requirements specified by the customer, including the requirements for delivery and post-delivery activities?
	b) Requirements not stated by the customer but necessary for specified or intended use, where known?
	c) Statutory and regulatory requirements related to the product?
	d) Any additional requirements determined by the organization?
EU	Vefiy that manufacturing maintains files containing or refer to the location of objective evidence establishing the safety and effectiveness of the device as required by Annex 1 of the MDD. Verify that the manufacturer followed a defined and effective process to establish and maintain a file containing documents defining product specifications and quality system requirements for each newa and existing type/modes of medical devices. Since the last audit, has the manufacturer introduced new products in the EU? Has the manufacturer followed a defined and effective process to obtain an approval from the Notified Body to CE mark a product prior to selling it in the EU? (does not apply to class I devices)

Doc. Reference	Adequate?	Stage I (clauses marked *)	Stage II

	REQUIREMENTS
USA	Verify that the firm has the appropriate marketing clearance [510(k)] or pre-market approval (PMA) if distributing the devices in the United States [21 CFR 807]. 21 CFR -807.81 When a pre-market notification is required: Each person who is required to register his establishment pursuant to 807.20 must submit a premarket notification submission to the Food and Drug Administration at least 90 days before he proposes to begin the introduction or delivery for introduction into interstate commerce for commercial distribution of a device intended for human use which meets any of the following criteria: (1) The device is being introduced into commercial distribution for the first time; that is, the device is not of the same type as, or is not substantially equivalent to, (i) a device in commercial distribution before May 1976 ,28, or (ii) a device introduced for commercial distribution after May ,28 1976, that has subsequently been reclassified into class I or II. (2) The device is being introduced into commercial distribution for the first time by a person required to register 21 CFR 814 – Premarket Approval; A Premarket approval is required for any FDA class III device that was not on the market (introduced or delivered for introduction into commerce for commercial distribution) before May ,28 1976, and is not substantially equivalent to a device on the market before May 1976 ,28, or to a device first marketed on, or after that date, which has been classified into class I or class II.
7.2.2 Review of requirements related to the product	
	Does the organization review the requirements related to the product?

Doc. Reference	Adequate?	Stage I (clauses marked *)	Stage II

	REQUIREMENTS
	Is this review conducted prior to the organization's commitment to supply a product to the customer (e.g. submission of tenders, acceptance of contracts or orders, acceptance of changes to contracts or orders)?
	Does the organization ensure that:
	a) Product requirements are defined and documented?
	b) Contract or order requirements differing from those previously expressed are resolved?
	c) The organization has the ability to meet the defined requirements?
	Are records of the results of the review and actions arising from the review maintained (see 4.2.4)?
	Where the customer provides no documented statement of requirement, are the customer requirements confirmed by the organization before acceptance?
	Where product requirements are changed, does the organization ensure that relevant documents are amended and that relevant personnel are made aware of the changed requirements?
7.2.3 Customer communication	
	Has the organization determined and implemented effective arrangements for communicating with customers in relation to:
	a) Product information?
	b) Enquiries, contracts or order handling, including amendments?
	c) Customer feedback, including customer complaints? (see 8.2.1)
	d) Advisory notices? (see 8.5.1)
7.3 Design and development	
7.3.1 Design and/or development planning	

Doc. Reference	Adequate?	Stage I (clauses marked *)	Stage II

	REQUIREMENTS
	Has the organization established documented procedures for design and development?
	Does the organization plan and control the design and development of product?
	During the design and development planning, does the organization determine:
	a) The design and development stages?
	b) The review, verification, validation and design transfer activities (see Note) that are appropriate at each design and development stage?
	c) The responsibilities and authorities for design and development?
	Does the organization manage the interfaces between different groups involved in design and development to ensure effective communication and clear assignment of responsibility?
	Is planning output documented, and updated as appropriate, as the design and development progresses? (See 4.2.3)
7.3.2 Design and development inputs	
	Have inputs relating to product requirements been determined and records maintained (see 4.2.4)?
	Do these inputs include:
	a) Functional, performance and safety requirements, according to the intended use?
	b) Applicable statutory and regulatory requirements?
	c) Where applicable, information derived from previous similar designs?
	d) Other requirements essential for design and development?
	e) Output(s) of risk management (see 7.1)?
	Are these inputs reviewed for adequacy and approved?

Doc. Reference	Adequate?	Stage I (clauses marked *)	Stage II

	REQUIREMENTS
	Are requirements complete, unambiguous and not in conflict with each other?
US	Verify that the design input procedures contain a mechanism for addressing incomplete, ambiguous, or conflicting requirements [21 CFR 820.30(c)].
7.3.3 Design and development outputs	
	Are the outputs of design and development provided in a form that enables verification against the design and development input, and is it approved prior to release?
	Do design and development outputs:
	a) meet the input requirements for design and development?
	b) Provide appropriate information for purchasing, production and for service provision?
	c) Contain or reference product acceptance criteria?
	d) Specify the characteristics of the product that are essential for its safe and proper use?
	Are records of the design and development outputs maintained (see 4.2.4)?
7.3.4 Design and development review	
	At suitable stages, are systematic reviews of design and development performed in accordance with planned arrangements (see 7.3.1):
	a) To evaluate the ability of the results of design and development to meet requirements?
	b) To identify any problems and propose necessary actions?
	Do participants in such reviews include representatives of functions concerned with the design and development stage(s) being reviewed, as well as other specialist personnel (see 5.5.1 and 6.2.1)?
	Are records of the results of the reviews and any necessary actions maintained (see 4.2.4)?

Doc. Reference	Adequate?	Stage I (clauses marked *)	Stage II

	REQUIREMENTS
US	Verify that procedures ensure that participants include representatives of all functions concerned with the design stage being reviewed and an individual(s) who does not have direct responsibility for the design stage being reviewed, as well as any specialists needed [21 CFR 820.30(e)].
EU	Does the supplier evaluate the need for risk analysis throughout the design process and maintain records of any risk analysis performed? (MDD Annex 1)
7.3.5 Design and development verification	
	Is verification performed in accordance with planned arrangements (see 7.3.1) to ensure that the design and development outputs have met the design and development input requirements?
	Are records of the results of the verification and any necessary actions maintained?
7.3.6 Design and development validation	
	Is design and development validation performed in accordance with planned arrangements (see 7.3.1) to ensure that the resulting product is capable of meeting the requirements for the specified application or intended use?
	Is validation completed prior to the delivery or implementation of the product (see Note 1)?
	Are records of the results of validation and any necessary actions maintained (see 4.2.4)?
	As part of design and development validation, does the organization perform clinical evaluations and/or evaluation of performance of the medical device, as required by national or regional regulations (see Note 2)?

Doc. Reference	Adequate?	Stage I (clauses marked *)	Stage II

	REQUIREMENTS
US	Verify that design validation has been performed on initial production units, lots, or batches, or their equivalents. When equivalent devices are used in the final validation, the manufacturer must document in detail how the device was manufactured and how the device is similar to and possibly different from initial production. When there are differences, the manufacturer must justify why design validation results are valid for the production units, lots, or batches. Verify that design validation includes testing of production units under actual or simulated use conditions [21 CFR 820.30(g)].
7.3.7 Control of design and development changes	
	Are design and development changes identified and records maintained?
	Are changes reviewed, verified, and validated, as appropriate, and approved before implementation?
	Does the review of design and development changes include evaluation of the effect of the changes on constituent parts and product already delivered?
	Are records of the results of the review of changes and any necessary actions maintained?
US	Verify that the firm obtained a new 510(k) or supplement to the pre-market approval if required [21 CFR 807].
EU	Do documented procedures identify the need to report essential changes to the Notified Body, (MDD Annex II, V, VI, 3.4)
7.4 Purchasing	
7.4.1 Purchasing process	
	Has the organization established documented procedures to ensure that purchased product conforms to specified purchase requirements?

Doc. Reference	Adequate?	Stage I (clauses marked *)	Stage II

	REQUIREMENTS
	Is the type and extent of control applied to the supplier and the purchased product dependent upon the effect of the purchased product on subsequent product realization or the final product?
	Does the organization evaluate and select suppliers based on their ability to supply product in accordance with the organization's requirements?
	Have criteria for selection, evaluation and re-evaluation been established?
	Are records of the results of evaluation and any necessary actions arising from the evaluation maintained (see 4.2.4)?
	Does purchasing information describe the product to be purchased, including where appropriate:
	a) Requirements for approval of product, procedures, processes and equipment?
	b) Requirements for qualification of personnel?
	c) Quality management system requirements?
	Does the organization ensure the adequacy of specified purchase requirements prior to their communication to the supplier?
	To the extent required for traceability given in 7.5.3.2, does the organization maintain relevant purchasing information, i.e. documents (see 4.2.3) and records (see 4.2.4)?
7.4.3 Verification of purchased product	
	Has the organization established and implemented the inspection or other activities necessary for ensuring that purchased product meets specified purchase requirements?
	Where the organization or its customer intends to perform verification at the supplier's premises, does the organization state the intended verification arrangements and method of product release in the purchasing information?
	Are records of the verification maintained (see 4.2.4)?

Doc. Reference	Adequate?	Stage I (clauses marked *)	Stage II

	REQUIREMENTS

7.5 Production and service provision

7.5.1 Control of production and service provision

7.5.1.1 General Requirements

	Does the organization plan and carry out production and service provision under controlled conditions?
	Do the controlled conditions include, as applicable:
	a) The availability of information that describes the characteristics of the product?
	b) The availability of documented procedures, documented requirements, work instructions, reference materials and reference measurement procedures as necessary?
	c) The use of suitable equipment?
	d) The availability and use of monitoring and measuring devices?
	e) The implementation of monitoring and measurement?
	f) The implementation of release, delivery and post-delivery activities?
	g) The implementation of defined operations for labeling and packaging?
	Does the organization establish and maintain a record (see 4.2.4) for each batch of medical devices that provides traceability to the extent specified in 7.5.3 and identifies the amount manufactured and amount approved for distribution?
	Is the batch record verified and approved?

Doc. Reference	Adequate?	Stage I (clauses marked *)	Stage II

	REQUIREMENTS
US	Verify that labeling is not released for storage or use until a designated individual has examined the labeling for accuracy. The release, including the date and signature of the individual performing the examination must be documented in the device history record (i.e. batch record) [21 CFR 820.120(b)]. Confirm that labeling is stored in a manner that provides proper identification and prevents mix-ups. Verify that labeling and packaging operations are controlled to prevent labeling mix-ups [21 CFR 820.120(c) and (d)]. Verify that the label and labeling used for each production unit, lot, or batch are documented in the batch record, as well as any control numbers used [21 CFR 820.120(e), 820.184(e)].

7.5.1.2 Control of production and service provision — Specific requirement

7.5.1.2.1 Cleanliness of product and contamination control

	Does the organization establish documented requirements for cleanliness of product if:
	a) Product is cleaned by the organization prior to sterilization and/or its use, or
	b) Product is supplied non-sterile to be subjected to a cleaning process prior to sterilization and/or its use, or
	c) Product is supplied to be used non-sterile and its cleanliness is of significance in use, or
	d) Process agents are to be removed from product during manufacture?
	If product is cleaned in accordance with a) or b) above, the requirements contained in 6.4 a) and 6.4 b) do not apply prior to the cleaning process.

7.5.1.2.2 Installation activities

Doc. Reference	Adequate?	Stage I (clauses marked *)	Stage II

	REQUIREMENTS
	If appropriate, does the organization establish documented requirements which contain acceptance criteria for installing and verifying the installation of the medical device?
	If the agreed customer requirements allow installation to be performed other than by the organization or its authorized agent, does the organization provide documented requirements for installation and verification?
	Are records of installation and verification performed by the organization or its authorized agent maintained (see 4.2.4)?
7.5.1.2.3 Servicing activities	
	If servicing is a specified requirement, does the organization establish documented procedures, work instructions and reference materials and reference measurement procedures, as necessary, for performing servicing activities and verifying that they meet the specified requirements?
	Are records of servicing activities carried out by the organization maintained (see 4.2.4)?
US	Verify that each manufacturer who receives a service report that represents an event that must be reported to FDA as a medical device report automatically considers the report a complaint [21 CFR 820.200(c)]. Confirm that service reports are documented and include the name of the device serviced, any device identification(s) and control number(s) used, and the date of service [21 CFR 820.200(d)].
7.5.1.3 Particular requirements for sterile medical devices	
	Does the organization maintain records of the process parameters for the sterilization process which was used for each sterilization batch (see 4.2.4)?
	Are sterilization records traceable to each production batch of medical devices (see 7.5.1.1)?
7.5.2 Validation of processes for production and service provision	

Doc. Reference	Adequate?	Stage I (clauses marked *)	Stage II

	REQUIREMENTS

7.5.2.1 General requirements	
	Does the organization validate any processes for production and service provision where the resulting output cannot be verified by subsequent monitoring or measurement? (this includes any processes where deficiencies become apparent only after the product is in use or the service has been delivered)
	Does validation demonstrate the ability of the processes to achieve planned results?
	Has the organization established arrangements for these processes including, as applicable:
	a) Defined criteria for review and approval of the processes?
	b) Approval of equipment and qualification of personnel?
	c) Use of specific methods and procedures?
	d) Requirements for records (see 4.2.4)?
	e) Re-validation?
	Has the organization established documented procedures for the validation of the application of computer software (and changes to such software and/or its application) for production and service provision that affect the ability of the product to conform to specified requirements?
	Are such software applications validated prior to initial use?
	Are records of validation maintained (see 4.2.4)?
US	Process validation is required for sterilization, aseptic processing, injection molding, and welding [21 CFR 820.75; preamble comment 143].
US	Confirm that the validation activities and results, including the date and signature of the individual approving the validation and where appropriate the major equipment validated, have been documented [21 CFR 820.75(a)].
7.5.2.2 Particular requirements for sterile medical devices	

Doc. Reference	Adequate?	Stage I (clauses marked *)	Stage II

	REQUIREMENTS
	Has the organization established documented procedures for the validation of sterilization processes?
	Are sterilization processes validated prior to initial use?
	Are records of validation of each sterilization process maintained (see 4.2.4)?
7.5.3 Identification and traceability	
7.5.3.1 Identification	
	Does the organization identify the product by suitable means throughout product realization and does the organization establish documented procedures for such product identification?
	Has the organization established documented procedures to ensure that medical devices returned to the organization are identified and distinguished from conforming product [see 6.4 d)]?
7.5.3.2 Traceability	
7.5.3.2.1 General	
	Has the organization established documented procedures for traceability?
	Do such procedures define the extent of product traceability and the records required (see 8.3 ,4.2.4 and 8.5)?
	Does the organization control and record the unique identification of the product, where traceability is a requirement (see 4.2.4)?
US	If a control number is required for traceability, confirm that such control number is on or accompanies the device throughout distribution [21 CFR 820.120(e)].

Doc. Reference	Adequate?	Stage I (clauses marked *)	Stage II

	REQUIREMENTS
EU	Does the manufacturer have procedures identifying the requirements of labeling and instructions for use as defined in MDD, Annex 1 point 13, and is regulations for CE marking included in these procedures. (MDD 3, Article 17 and Annex 12).
	Are language requirements defined in procedures for the information identified in MDD, Annex 1point 13 for the applicable markets.
7.5.3.2.2 Particular requirements for active implantable medical devices and	
	In defining the records required for traceability, does the organization include records of all components, materials and work environment conditions, if these could cause the medical device not to satisfy its specified requirements?
	Does the organization require that its agents or distributors maintain records of the distribution of medical devices to allow traceability and that such records be available for inspection?
	Are records of the name and address of the shipping package consignee maintained (see 4.2.4)?
US	Verify that the manufacturer has implemented a tracking system for devices for which the manufacturer has received a tracking order from FDA. The tracking system must ensure the manufacturer is able to track the device to the end-user. The manufacturer must conduct periodic audits of the tracking system [21 CFR 821].
7.5.3.3 Status identification	
	Does the organization identify the product status with respect to monitoring and measurement requirements?
	Is the identification of product status maintained throughout production, storage, installation and servicing of the product to ensure that only product that has passed the required inspections and tests (or released under an authorized concession) is dispatched, used or installed?

Doc. Reference	Adequate?	Stage I (clauses marked *)	Stage II

e medical devices

	REQUIREMENTS

	7.5.4 Customer property
	Does the organization exercise care with customer property while it is under the organization's control or being used by the organization?
	Does the organization identify, verify, protect and safeguard customer property provided for use or incorporation into the product?
	If any customer property is lost, damaged, or otherwise found to be unsuitable for use, is this reported to the customer and are records maintained (see 4.2.4)?
	7.5.5 Preservation of product
	Has the organization established documented procedures or documented work instructions for preserving the conformity of product during internal processing and delivery to the intended destination?
	Does this preservation include identification, handling, packaging, storage and protection, and also apply to the constituent parts of a product?
	Has the organization established documented procedures or documented work instructions for the control of product with a limited shelf-life or requiring special storage conditions?
	Are such special storage conditions controlled and recorded (see 4.2.4)?

Doc. Reference	Adequate?	Stage I (clauses marked *)	Stage II

	REQUIREMENTS
US	Confirm that the manufacturer established and maintains procedures that describe the methods for authorizing receipt from and dispatch to storage areas and stock rooms [21 CFR 150(b)]. Verify that the manufacturer established and maintains procedures for control and distribution of finished devices to ensure that only those devices approved for release are distributed and that purchase orders are reviewed to ensure ambiguities and errors are resolved before devices are released for distribution [21 CFR 820.160(a)].
7.6 Control of monitoring and measuring devices	
	Does the organization determine monitoring and measuring to be undertaken and the monitoring and measuring devices needed to provide evidence of conformity of product to determined requirements (guide reference 7.2.1)?
	Has the organization established documented procedures to ensure that monitoring and measurement can be carried out and are carried out in a manner that is consistent with the monitoring and measurement requirements?
	Where necessary to ensure valid results, is measuring equipment:
	a) Calibrated or verified at specified intervals, or prior to use, against measurement standards traceable to international or national measurement standards; where no such standards exist, is the basis used for calibration or verification recorded?
	b) Adjusted or re-adjusted as necessary?
	c) Identified to enable the calibration status to be determined?
	d) Safeguarded from adjustments that would invalidate the measurement result?
	e) Protected from damage and deterioration during handling, maintenance and storage?

Doc. Reference	Adequate?	Stage I (clauses marked *)	Stage II

	REQUIREMENTS
	Does the organization assess and record the validity of the previous measuring results when the equipment is found not to conform to requirements?
	Does the organization take appropriate action on the equipment and any product affected?
	Are records of the results of calibration and verification maintained (see 4.2.4)?
	When used in the monitoring and measurement of specified requirements, is the ability of computer software to satisfy the intended application confirmed prior to initial use and reconfirmed as necessary ?
8 Measurement, analysis and improvement	
8.1 General	
	Does the organization plan and implement the monitoring, measurement, analysis and improvement processes needed:
	a) To demonstrate conformity of the product?
	b) To ensure conformity of the quality management system?
	c) To maintain the effectiveness of the quality management system?
	Does this include determination of applicable methods, including statistical techniques, and the extent of their use?
US	Where appropriate, verify the organization has established and maintained procedures for identifying valid statistical techniques required for establishing, controlling , and verifying the acceptability of process capability and product characteristics [21 CFR 820.250(a)].
8.2 Monitoring and measurement	
8.2.1 Feedback	
	As one of the measurements of the performance of the quality management system, does the organization monitor information relating to whether the organization has met customer requirements?

Doc. Reference	Adequate?	Stage I (clauses marked *)	Stage II

	REQUIREMENTS
	Have the methods for obtaining and using this information been determined?
	Has the organization established a documented procedure for a feedback system [see 7.2.3 c)] to provide early warning of quality problems and for input into the corrective and preventive action processes (see 8.5.2 and 8.5.3)?
	If national or regional regulations require the organization to gain experience from the post-production phase, does the review of this experience form part of the feedback system (see 8.5.1)?
Canada	Verify that the manufacturer maintains records of reported problems related to the performance characteristics or safety of a device, including any consumer complaints received by the manufacturer after the device was first sold in Canada, and all actions taken by the manufacturer in response to the problems referred to in t hecomplaints [CMDR Section 57]. Verify that the manufacturer has established and implemented documented procedures that will enable it to carry out an effective and timely investigation of the problems reports through the customer complaints, andto carry out an effective and timely recall of the device [CMDR Section 58].
Japan	Confirm that the personnel operating the Registered Manufacturing Site has determined and implemented effective arrangements for communicating with the Japanese Marketing Authorization Holder in relation to customer feedback, including customer complaints, and advisory notices [MHLW MO29 :169].

Doc. Reference	Adequate?	Stage I (clauses marked *)	Stage II

	REQUIREMENTS
US	Verify procedures have been defined, documented, and implemented for receiving, reviewing, and evaluating complaints by a formally designated unit. Procedures must ensure that: (1) All complaints are processed in a uniform and timely manner (2) Oral complaints are documented upon receipt (3) Complaints are evaluated to determine whether the complaint represents an event which is required to be reported to FDA
	Each manufacturer must review and evaluate all complaints to determine whether an investigation is necessary. When no investigation is made, the manufacturer must maintain a record that includes the reason no investigation was made and the name of the individual responsible for the decision not to investigate. Any complaint of the failure of the device, labeling, or packaging to meet any of its specifications must be reviewed, evaluated, and investigated, unless such investigation has already been made for a similar complaint and another investigation is not necessary. Any complaint that represents an event which must be reported to FDA must be promptly reviewed, evaluated, and investigated by a designated individual(s) and must be maintained in a separate portion of the complaint files or otherwise clearly identified.
	When the manufacturer's formally designated unit is located at a site separate from the manufacturing establishment, the investigated complaint(s) and the record(s) of investigation must be reasonably accessible to the manufacturing establishment [21 CFR 820.198].

Doc. Reference	Adequate?	Stage I (clauses marked *)	Stage II

	REQUIREMENTS

8.2.2 Internal audit	
	Does the organization conduct internal audits at planned intervals to determine whether the quality management system
	a) Conforms to the planned arrangements (see 7.1), to the requirements of this International Standard and to the quality management system requirements established by the organization?
	b) Is effectively implemented and maintained?
	Is an audit programme planned, taking into consideration the status and importance of the processes and areas to be audited, as well as the results of previous audits?
	Are the audit criteria, scope, frequency and methods defined?
	Does selection of auditors and conduct of audits ensure objectivity and impartiality of the audit process (e.g. auditors shall not audit their own work)?
	Are the responsibilities and requirements for planning and conducting audits, and for reporting results and maintaining records (see 4.2.4) defined in a documented procedure?
	Does management responsible for the area being audited ensure that actions are taken without undue delay to eliminate detected nonconformities and their causes?
	Do follow-up activities include the verification of the actions taken and the reporting of verification results? (see 8.5.2)
US	Verify that resources include the assignment of trained personnel to meet the requirements of 21 CFR Part 820, including management, performance of work, assessment activities, and internal quality audits [21 CFR 820.20(b)(2)].
8.2.3 Measurement and monitoring of processes	

Doc. Reference	Adequate?	Stage I (clauses marked *)	Stage II

	REQUIREMENTS
	Does the organization apply suitable methods for monitoring and, where applicable, measurement of the quality management system processes?
	Do these methods demonstrate the ability of the processes to achieve planned results?
	When planned results are not achieved, is correction and corrective action taken, as appropriate, to ensure conformity of the product?
US	Verify that the manufacturer has established and maintains procedures for identifying valid statistical techniques required for establishing, controlling and verifying the acceptability of process capability and product characteristics, where appropriate [21 CFR 820.250(a)].
8.2.4 Monitoring and measurement of product	
8.2.4.1 General requirements	
	Does the organization monitor and measure the characteristics of the product to verify that product requirements have been met?
	Is this carried out at appropriate stages of the product realization process in accordance with the planned arrangements (see 7.1) and documented procedures (see 7.5.1.1)?
	Is evidence of conformity with the acceptance criteria maintained?
	Do records indicate the person(s) authorizing release of the product (see 4.2.4)?
	Does the organization ensure that product release and service delivery do not proceed until the planned arrangements (see 7.1) have been satisfactorily completed?

Doc. Reference	Adequate?	Stage I (clauses marked *)	Stage II

	REQUIREMENTS
US	Verify that the manufacturer establishes and maintains procedures to ensure that sampling methods are adequate for their intended use and ensure that when changes occur, the sampling plans are reviewed [21 CFR 820.250(b)].
	8.2.4.2 Particular requirement for active implantable medical devices and in
	Does the organization record (see 4.2.4) the identity of personnel performing any inspection or testing?
	8.3 Control of nonconforming product
	Does the organization ensure that product which does not conform to product requirements is identified and controlled to prevent its unintended use or delivery?
	Are the controls and related responsibilities and authorities for dealing with nonconforming product defined in a documented procedure?
	Does the organization deal with nonconforming product by one or more of the following ways?
	a) By taking action to eliminate the detected nonconformity
	b) By authorizing its use, release or acceptance under concession
	c) By taking action to preclude its original intended use or application
	Does the organization ensure that nonconforming product is accepted by concession only if regulatory requirements are met?
	Are records of the identity of the person(s) authorizing the concession maintained (see 4.2.4)?
	Are records of the nature of nonconformities and any subsequent actions taken, including concessions obtained maintained (see 4.2.4)?
	When nonconforming product is corrected, is it subject to re-verification to demonstrate conformity to the requirements?

Doc. Reference	Adequate?	Stage I (clauses marked *)	Stage II
nedical devices			

	REQUIREMENTS
	When nonconforming product is detected after delivery or use has started, does the organization take action appropriate to the effects, or potential effects, of the nonconformity?
	If product needs to be reworked (one or more times), does the organization document the rework process in a work instruction that has undergone the same authorization and approval procedure as the original work instruction?
	Prior to authorization and approval of the work instruction, is a determination of any adverse effect of the rework upon product made and documented (see 4.2.3 and 7.5.1)?
US	Confirm that the evaluation of non-conforming product includes a determination of the need for an investigation and notification of the persons or organizations responsible for the nonconformance. The evaluation and any investigation must be documented [21 CFR 820.90(a)].
8.4 Analysis of data	
	Does the organization establish documented procedures to determine, collect and analyse appropriate data to demonstrate the suitability and effectiveness of the quality management system and to evaluate if improvement of the effectiveness of the quality management system can be made?
	Does this include data generated as a result of monitoring and measurement and from other relevant sources?
	Does the analysis of data provide information relating to:
	a) Feedback (see 8.2.1)?
	b) Conformity to product requirements? (See 7.2.1)
	c) Characteristics and trends of processes and products including opportunities for preventive action?
	d) Suppliers?
	Are records of the results of the analysis of data maintained (see 4.2.4)?

Doc. Reference	Adequate?	Stage I (clauses marked *)	Stage II

	REQUIREMENTS	

8.5 Improvement		
8.5.1 General		
	Does the organization identify and implement any changes necessary to ensure and maintain the continued suitability and effectiveness of the quality management system through the use of the quality policy, quality objectives, audit results, analysis of data, corrective and preventive actions and management review?	
	Does the organization establish documented procedures for the issue and implementation of advisory notices and are these procedures capable of being implemented at any time?	
US	Verify that the manufacturer has a process in place to notify FDA in the event of actions concerning device corrections and removals and to maintain records of those corrections and removals. [21 CFR 806: Medical Devices; Reports of Corrections and Removals]	
EU	Are the procedures for Vigilance reporting in conformance with MDD Annex II, V, and VI (MEDDEV 1ʼ-2.12)	
	Are records of all customer complaint investigations maintained (see 4.2.4)?	
	If investigation determines that the activities outside the organization contributed to the customer complaint, is relevant information exchanged between the organizations involved (see 4.1)?	
	If any customer complaint is not followed by corrective and/ or preventive action, is the reason authorized (see 5.5.1) and recorded (see 4.2.4)?	
US	Verify that information related to quality problems or nonconforming product is disseminated to those directly responsible for assuring the quality of such product or the prevention of such problems [21 CFR 820.100(a)(6)].	

Doc. Reference	Adequate?	Stage I (clauses marked *)	Stage II

	REQUIREMENTS
	If national or regional regulations require notification of adverse events that meet specific reporting criteria, does the organization establish documented procedures to such notification to regulatory authorities?
US	Determine whether the manufacturer has developed a process for reporting to FDA incidents involving device-related deaths, serious injuries, and reportable malfunctions that occur within and outside the United States if the same or similar device is marketed to the United States. Confirm that the manufacturer has developed, maintained, and implemented written medical device reporting (MDR) procedures compliant with the requirements of: [21 CFR 803: Medical Device Reporting]
EU	Are procedures for the reporting of recall to the relevant competent authority and the NB compliant? (MDD, Annex II, V, VI, 3.1)
8.5.2 Corrective action	
	Does the organization take action to eliminate the cause of nonconformities in order to prevent recurrence and are corrective actions appropriate to the effects of the nonconformities encountered?

Doc. Reference	Adequate?	Stage I (clauses marked *)	Stage II

	REQUIREMENTS
	Has a documented procedure been established to define requirements for:
	a) Reviewing nonconformities (including customer complaints)?
	b) Determining the causes of nonconformities?
	c) Evaluating the need for action to ensure that nonconformities do no recur?
	d) Determining and implementing action needed, including, if appropriate, updating documentation (see 4.2)?
	e) Recording of the results of any investigation and of action taken (see 4.2.4)?
	f) Reviewing the corrective action taken and its effectiveness?
US	Verify that procedures are in place for verifying or validating the corrective and preventive action to ensure the action is effective and does not adversely affect the finished device [21 CFR 820.100(a)(4)]. Verify procedures ensure that information related to quality problems or nonconforming product is disseminated to those directly responsible for assuring the quality of such product or the prevention of problems [21 CFR 820.100(a)(6)]. Confirm procedures provide for the submission of relevant information on identified quality problems, as well as corrective and preventive actions, for management review [21 CFR 820.100(a)(7)].
8.5.3 Preventive action	
	Does the organization determine action to eliminate the causes of potential nonconformities in order to prevent their occurrence and are preventive actions appropriate to the effects of the potential problems?

Doc. Reference	Adequate?	Stage I (clauses marked *)	Stage II

	REQUIREMENTS
	Has a documented procedure been established to define requirements for:
	a) Determining potential nonconformities and their causes?
	b) Evaluating the need for action to prevent occurrence of nonconformities?
	c) Determining and implementing action needed?
	d) Recording of the results of any investigations and of action taken (see 4.2.4)?
	e) Reviewing preventive action taken and its effectiveness?

Doc. Reference	Adequate?	Stage I (clauses marked *)	Stage II

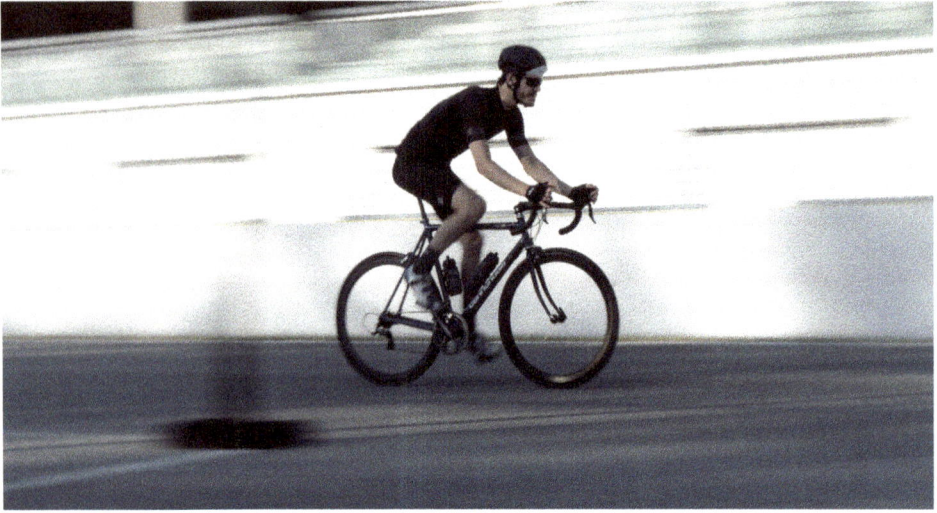

The system is working for you (the system is fully integrated along your processes and eases your operations).

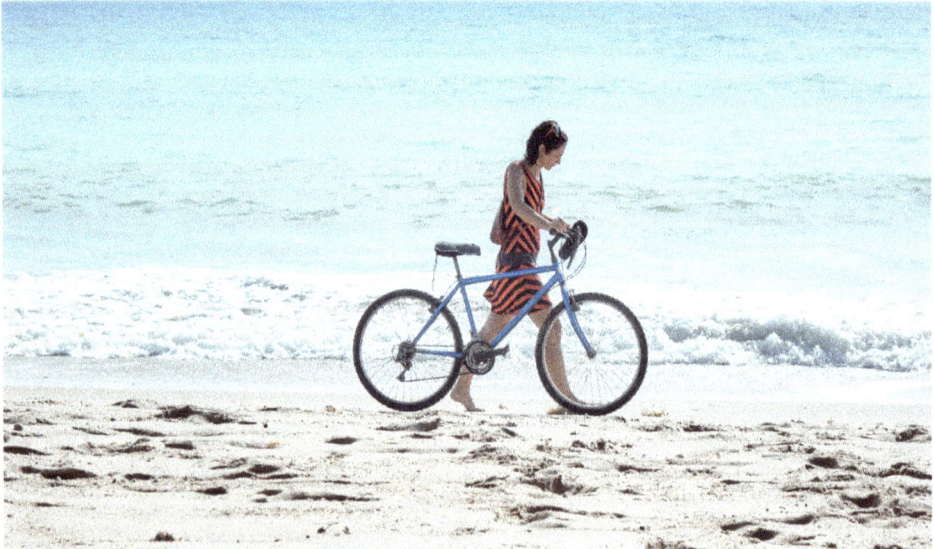

You are working for the system
(the system is beside your operations and looks as an additional burden.)

Advice for manufacturers planning certification

Firstly, you should confirm that the device(s) your company manufactures can be defined as a medical device under ISO 13485 standards; or, if you provide a medical device service, that your service is related to a product defined as a medical device. Getting ISO 13485 certification is challenging and requires commitment so, secondly, it's important that your leadership team confirms that holding the certification will add value to your company, meet its business objectives and support its strategy. While holding the full certification is not strictly necessary, as your company can still conform to and benefit from ISO 13485 standards without being externally certified, it does clearly demonstrate to all stakeholders that you comply with its requirements.

If you do want to become independently certified there are two phases; the first covers documentation, while the second implements your quality management system and audits it. You must carry out phase two within six months of completing phase one.

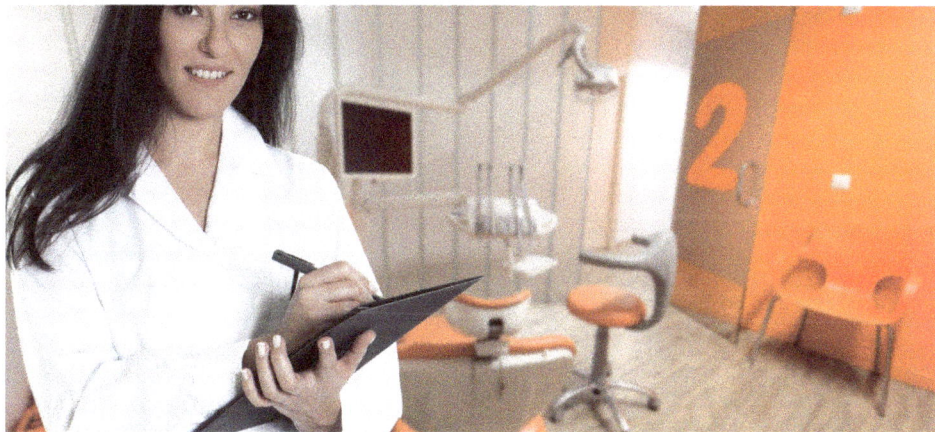

ISO 13485 certification costs

For companies who wish to be fully ISO 13485 certified, there are associated costs for external, independent certification. Although you may be under cost pressure, it's important to work with an independent auditor who will add real value to your company during the certification process. In this highly regulated industry, choose a reputable auditing company with extensive expertise rather than one that enables you to gain certification at the lowest price.

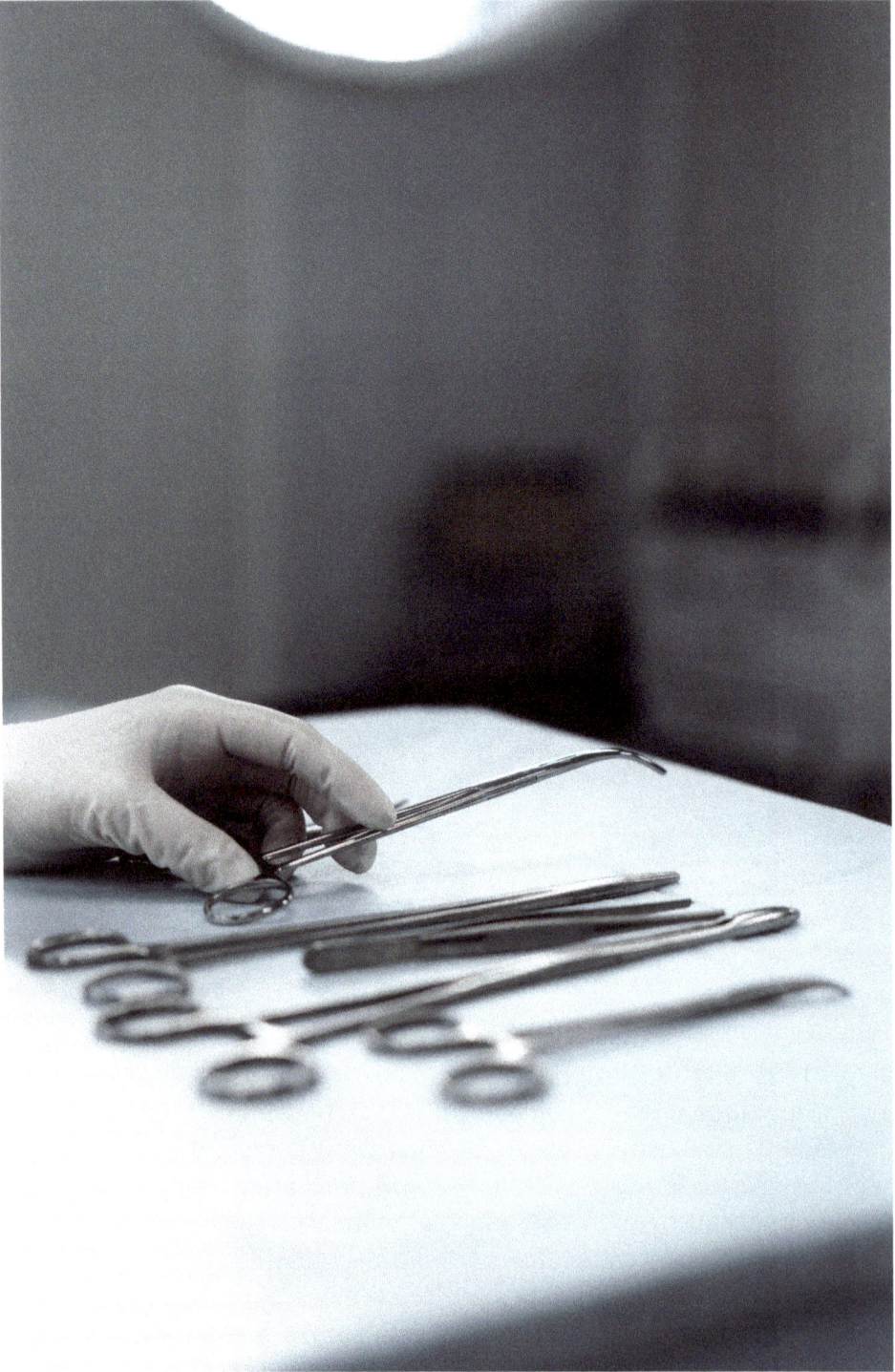

Bibliography

Bibliography:

Astrini, N. (2018). ISO 9001 and performance: a method review. Total Quality Management & Business Excellence, doi: 10.1080/14783363.2018.1524293.

Asadi,J, Easy ISo 13485:2016, Silosa Consulting Group, 2022

Bou-Llusar, J. C., Escrig-Tena, A. B., Roca-Puig, V., & Beltra´n-Martı´n, I. (2005). To what extent do enablers explain results in the EFQM excellence model? International Journal of Quality & Reliability Management, 22(44), 337-353.

Chatzoglou, P., Chatzoudes, D., & Kipraios, N. (2015). The impact of ISO 9000 certification on firms' financial performance. International Journal of Operations and Production Management, 35(1), 145-174. https://doi.org/10.1108/IJOPM-07-2012-0387

Definition of the terms "medical device" and "in vitro diagnostic (IVD) medical device". Global Harmonization Task Force;

Guidelines for regulatory auditing of quality systems of medical device manufacturers – Part 1: general requirements

Global Medical Devices Nomenclature System (GMDN) [website] (https://www. gmdnagency.org, accessed 2 February 2017).

FDA website address: fda.gov

Gigante, N., & Ziantoni, S. (2015). L'edizione 2015 della norma ISO 9001, 2015. Retrieved from:https://www.accredia.it/app/uploads/2015/12/6050_5_L__700_edizione_2015_della_norma_ISO_9001___Arch__Gigante__Dr__Ziantoni.pdf

ISO (2015a). ISO 9001 - Quality management systems – requirements. Geneva: International Organization for Standardization.

Role of standards in the assessment of medical devices. Global Harmonization Task Force; 2008 ISO (2018). ISO 19011 - Guidelines for auditing management systems quality management systems. Geneva: International Organization for Standardization.

ISO (2019). ISO 9000 Family - Quality Management. Retrieved from: https://www.iso.org/home.html.

Wilson, J. P., & Campbell, L. (2018). ISO 9001:2015: the evolution and convergence of quality management and knowledge management for competitive advantage. Total Quality Management and Business Excellence, pp. 1-16. https://doi.org/10.1080/ 14783363.2018.1445965

ONLINE
EDUCATION

START YOUR ONLINE COURSE NOW AFTER YOU HAVE COMPLETED READING THIS BOOK, DO YOUR QUIZZES AND RECEIVE YOUR INTERNATIONAL TRAINING CERTIFICATE OF :

ISO 13485

JOIN US AT: **MDSAP**

www.ISCASC.com